WORKBOOK FOR QUALITY MAMMOGRAPHY

Second Edition

D1232723

WORKBOOK FOR QUALITY MAMMOGRAPHY

Second Edition

CAROLYN KIMME-SMITH, PhD
Associate Professor
Iris Cantor Center for Breast Imaging
Department of Radiological Sciences
UCLA School of Medicine
Jonsson Comprehensive Cancer Center
Los Angeles, California

LAWRENCE W. BASSETT, MD
Professor of Breast Imaging
Iris Cantor Center for Breast Imaging
Department of Radiological Sciences
UCLA School of Medicine
Jonsson Comprehensive Cancer Center
Los Angeles, California

RICHARD H. GOLD, MD
Professor and Executive Vice Chairman
Department of Radiological Sciences
UCLA School of Medicine
Los Angeles, California

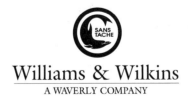

Williams & Wilkins
A WAVERLY COMPANY
BALTIMORE • PHILADELPHIA • LONDON • PARIS • BANGKOK
BUENOS AIRES • HONG KONG • MUNICH • SYDNEY • TOKYO • WROCLAW

Editor: Victoria M. Vaughn
Managing Editor: Grace E. Miller
Production Coordinator: Raymond E. Reter
Copy Editor: Therese Grundl
Designer: Wilma E. Rosenberger
Illustration Planner: Ray Lowman
Typesetter: University Graphics, Inc., York, Pennsylvania
Manufacturing: R.R. Donnelley & Sons, Crawfordsville, Indiana

Copyright © 1997 Williams & Wilkins

351 West Camden Street
Baltimore, Maryland 21201-2436 USA

Rose Tree Corporate Center
1400 North Providence Road
Building II, Suite 5025
Media, Pennsylvania 19063-2043 USA

Accurate indications, adverse reactions and dosage schedules for drugs are provided in this book, but it is possible that they may change. The reader is urged to review the package information data of the manufacturers of the medications mentioned.

Printed in the United States of America

First Edition, 1992

Library of Congress Cataloging-in-Publication Data

Kimme-Smith, Carolyn.
    Workbook for quality mammography / Carolyn Kimme-Smith, Lawrence W. Bassett, Richard H. Gold.
        p.   cm.
    Includes bibliographical references and index.
    ISBN 0-683-04612-8
    1. Breast—Radiography.   I. Bassett, Lawrence W. (Lawrence Wayne), 1942–   .
    II. Gold, Richard H.   III. Title.
    [DNLM: 1. Mammography—methods.   2. Mammography—instrumentation.
    3. Quality Control. WP 815 K49w 1997]
    RG493.5.R33K54   1997
    618.1'907572—dc20
    DNLM/DLC
    for Library of Congress   96-2980
                                                                      CIP

The publishers have made every effort to trace the copyright holders for borrowed material. If they have inadvertently overlooked any, they will be pleased to make the necessary arrangements at the first opportunity.

To purchase additional copies of this book, call our customer service department at **(800) 638-0672** or fax orders to **(800) 447-8438**. For other book services, including chapter reprints and large quantity sales, ask for the Special Sales department.

Canadian customers should call **(800) 268-4178** or fax **(905) 470-6780**. For all other calls originating outside of the United States, please call **(410) 528-4223** or fax **(410) 528-8550**.

Visit Williams & Wilkins on the Internet: **http://www.wwilkins.com** or contact our customer service department at **custserv@wwilkins.com**. Williams & Wilkins customer service representatives are available from 8:30 am to 6:00 pm, EST, Monday through Friday, for telephone access.

96 97 98 99 00
1 2 3 4 5 6 7 8 9 10

PREFACE TO THE SECOND EDITION

In the past 5 years the quality of mammography in the United States has significantly improved. Both the American College of Radiology's Mammography Accreditation Program and the National Mammography Quality Standards Act have contributed to this advance. Increased requirements for mammography education of radiology residents and for continuing medical education in mammography for radiologists have led to a higher yield of carcinoma detection. In the past 5 years, for biopsies performed on women with nonpalpable mammographically detected abnormalities, these yields have risen from 20 to 45% at some breast centers. The specialized training now required of radiologic technologists and medical physicists has helped them to consistently achieve higher quality mammograms.

Since publication of the first edition of this workbook, mammography equipment has been introduced that contains new anode and filter materials, new breast positioning improvements, innovative grid systems, and automatic exposure control systems that presample the breast. In addition to the upright add-on stereotactic devices for needle biopsy of lesions, dedicated prone stereotactic units have become widely available.

Most mammography facilities now perform breast ultrasound examinations. Radiologic technologists often perform ultrasonography in the mammography facility, and they may need training in the use of ultrasound equipment. We have included a chapter that describes ultrasound equipment most commonly used for breast examinations and methods to obtain high quality images.

Digital mammography is used in commercially available stereotactic core biopsy units. Several manufacturers are developing whole breast digital systems. Chapter 13 describes the differences between screen/film and digital mammography and the required technique changes for digital mammography.

The Mammography Quality Standards Act mandates adherence to quality control. The Food and Drug Administration has developed regulations specifying the quality assurance procedures and protocols with which mammography facilities must comply. The American College of Radiology provides manuals describing these quality control protocols as well as methods for breast positioning. Therefore, chapters on these procedures have been replaced with Chapters 3, "Evaluation of Clinical Imaging," and 11, "Quality Control." The new material emphasizes identification of problems and problem solving.

All original chapters from the first edition have been revised. All of the review questions have been replaced, and self-evaluation continues to be an important component of this workbook.

CAROLYN KIMME-SMITH
LAWRENCE W. BASSETT
RICHARD H. GOLD

PREFACE TO THE FIRST EDITION

Mammography screening of asymptomatic women leads to the detection of breast cancer at an earlier stage than can be accomplished when mammography is performed on women who already have breast symptoms. Cancers detected by mammography usually are smaller than those found by physical examination. Occult cancers often consist of clusters of microcalcifications or masses less than 0.5 cm in diameter. The imaging excellence required for screening has led to an increased awareness of the need for education in mammography quality control (QC). Although this book includes information about specific QC tests, it is designed primarily to teach radiologists and technologists to recognize the differences between mammograms of high quality and those that are less than optimal. The performance of routine QC procedures does not always identify faults in equipment, breast positioning, or x-ray technique as readily as breast image analysis by a well-trained radiologist or technologist. This self-teaching workbook not only shows how to recognize a high quality mammogram but also demonstrates how to correct inadequate image quality. In addition to describing tests to determine the causes of poor image quality, common practical problems that relate to mammography x-ray equipment, image processors, and image receptors are discussed.

Each chapter contains a review of basic concepts illustrated by radiographs and drawings. Technical faults in actual mammograms illustrate the workbook section of each chapter. The following text then describes how to diagnose and cure each technical problem. Because the eye must be trained to recognize good and poor quality mammography, more than half of this workbook consists of mammography images. Each chapter contains a short quiz and a list of published references selected not only to substantiate the text but also to augment it. The reference is followed by a short annotation related to its contents. Each chapter ends with a summarizing flowchart that lists the concepts covered and their interrelationships. Fifty multiple choice questions designed for board review and certification examinations are located at the end of the book. The answers to the fifty questions are referenced to pages in this workbook.

We have been diagnosing technical problems, teaching how to avoid and correct them, calibrating equipment, and answering questions about mammography QC for many years. This book is a compilation of that experience. We hope that our text will enlighten and encourage the reader to obtain images of the highest possible quality for breast cancer detection.

CAROLYN KIMME-SMITH
LAWRENCE W. BASSETT
RICHARD H. GOLD

CONTENTS

1

UNIQUE REQUIREMENTS OF MAMMOGRAPHY

Mammogra   ·⸱⸱ally difficult examination. This
is partly b   ⸱⸱⸱⸱⸱ent is used,
rigorous c
radiologic
meet spe
types of
quire th
and ima
radiogr
optical
Radio§   y
must   n.
Mam   on
(a cl   na-
lign⸱   na-
lign⸱   e of
sin⸱   ffer-
en   s ad-
ec   either
c⸱   ⸱e en-
l⸱   ⸱ mag-
⸱   ⸱oft-tis-
                                                          ⸱ontrast
                                                          ⸱nces in
                                                          ⸱ tissue,
                                                          y an in-

spe⸱⸱⸱   ⸱ a narrow
⸱its use spe-
cial anodes with a ⸱⸱⸱⸱   (Mo). Many
units now combine these Mo anodes w⸱⸱⸱ ⸱odium (Rh)
filtration to change the beam spectrum. Two manufacturers also offer Rh anodes or tungsten (W) anodes for
mammography in addition to the Mo anode. General radiography W anodes have a broad energy spectrum and
operate most efficiently above 70 kVp, whereas Mo
anodes produce photons predominantly in the 16- to
19-keV range. When 26 kVp is selected for a mammography technique, most of the photon energy is in the

16- to 19-keV range, although some output from 20- to
26-keV occurs because of bremsstrahlung. Because low-
density masses need to be seen, the lower energy range
is critical in mammography. Rh produces photons near
23 keV because of its photoelectric response and is recommended for large or glandular breasts. In addition to
kVp, anode, and filter composition, there are many other
factors that affect contrast, and these will be explored in
Chapter 7.

SPATIAL RESOLUTION

Spatial resolution is as important as contrast resolution.
Mammography screen/film combinations are designed to
such critical standards that high contrast line pair test objects can be imaged with greater precision using mammography equipment than with most available x-ray
equipment. Because of its smaller focal spot and lower
kVp requirements, the output of mammography x-ray
tubes is much lower than that of general purpose x-ray
tubes. The 2- or 3-second exposures sometimes needed
to penetrate large breasts may result in motion unsharpness, which degrades spatial resolution. The use of Rh
or W anodes reduces this problem by reducing exposure
time. Spatial resolution can be affected by the geometry
of the mammography equipment as well as by the particular image receptor used. Resolution is discussed in
Chapters 6 and 8.

PENETRATION

Because of the Mo anode, with its small focal spot and
low kVp, the photon flux from a mammography x-ray
tube is less than that from a general radiography x-ray
tube. Greater photon flux is needed at the thickest part
of the breast, near the chest wall, rather than at the nipple. To obtain uniform breast exposure and to ensure
penetration near the chest wall, the cathode side of the
x-ray tube is located at the chest wall side of the breast
to allow the heel effect to compensate for poor photon
flux. In addition, taut breast compression is applied during the exposure to even out the breast thickness and to
decrease overall thickness. To improve contrast, grids are

necessary for very dense or thick breasts that produce more scattered radiation than fatty, thin breasts. Proper screen film selection and film development can also help improve optical density exposure and contrast by increasing image receptor speed to compensate for a low-powered x-ray unit or for dense breasts. Rh and W anode options, as well as the use of a Mo anode with a Rh filter, increase penetration while reducing radiation dose. Chapter 5 (concerning automatic exposure control adjustment for thick breasts) contains many examples in which penetration is discussed.

RADIATION DOSE

Mammographic dose continues to be a concern. Doses should be as low as possible while being consistent with good image quality. Radiation dose in mammography is affected by many factors, including the speed of the screen/film combination, anode/filter selection, film processing, generator and tube output, compression, and number of "retakes." Indeed, the mean glandular dose for a single image of a 4-cm thick compressed breast can vary from 50 to 200 mrad! The quality of digital mammograms will be highly dependent on the exposure needed to maintain a high ratio of information compared with noise in the image. Although background optical density can be manipulated digitally, the quality of the image will depend on the exposure used to produce it. Chapters 6–9 include material on radiation dose. Chapter 11 is primarily concerned with dose measurement and dose reduction.

REGULATORY ISSUES

The Mammography Quality Standards Act mandates quality mammography. The American College of Radiology mammography quality control manuals describe the performance of quality control procedures and positioning. The manuals do not show many of the artifacts and positioning errors that may occur. Chapter 3, "Evaluation of Clinical Images," provides instruction in evaluating clinical images for positioning and technical deficiencies and how to recognize artifacts in the mammographic image. Chapter 11, "Evaluation for Quality Control," describes possible pitfalls in compliance with Food and Drug Administration regulations and provides methods to improve the efficiency of the required record keeping.

Suggested Readings

Bassett LW, Gold RH, Kimme-Smith C. History of the technical development of mammography. In: Haus AG, Yaffe MJ, eds. Syllabus: a categorical course in physics. Technical aspects of breast imaging, 3rd ed. Radiological Society of North America 80th Annual Meeting, Nov 27–Dec 2, 1994.

   The syllabus as a whole, and this introductory article in particular, are highly recommended as background material. The editors have assembled an international panel of authors.

Bushberg JT, Siebert JA, Leidholdt EM Jr, Boone JM. Mammography. In: The essential physics of medical imaging. Baltimore: Williams & Wilkins, 1994:209–237.

   The instrumentation and physics of mammography are briefly and intensely summarized. It is recommended as a supplement to this workbook, consistent with the philosophy that two teachers are better than one.

Hendrick RE. Quality assurance in mammography: accreditation, legislation and compliance with quality control standards. Radiol Clin North Am 1992;30:243–255.

   This report describes the history of the American College of Radiology mammography accreditation program and its results as of 1991. The emergence of the Mammography Quality Standards Act and its goals are also described.

PROBLEM 1

This mammogram is correctly positioned and exposed, but the image was re-taken. Why did the technologist reject this mammogram? You may have to look at the retake ("Solution 1") to answer.

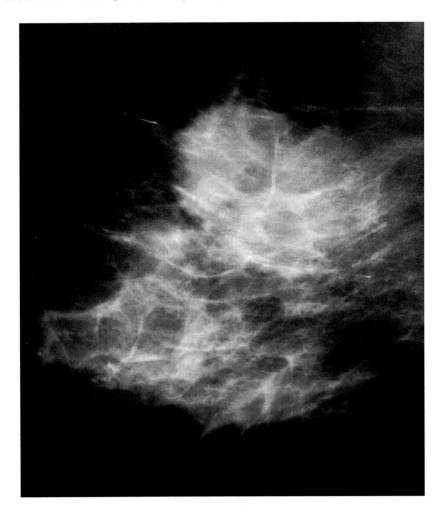

SOLUTION 1

The patient moved during the 2-sec exposure. Although the focal spot on this unit is small, exposures are long and motion often results.

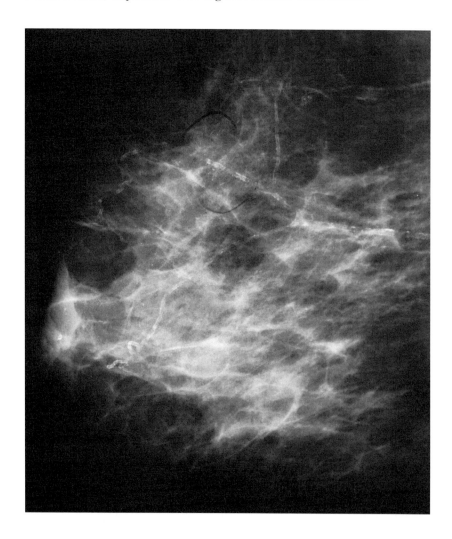

PROBLEM 2

What is the light band at the chest wall edge of the film? The physicist says the x-ray field covers the screen/film cassette.

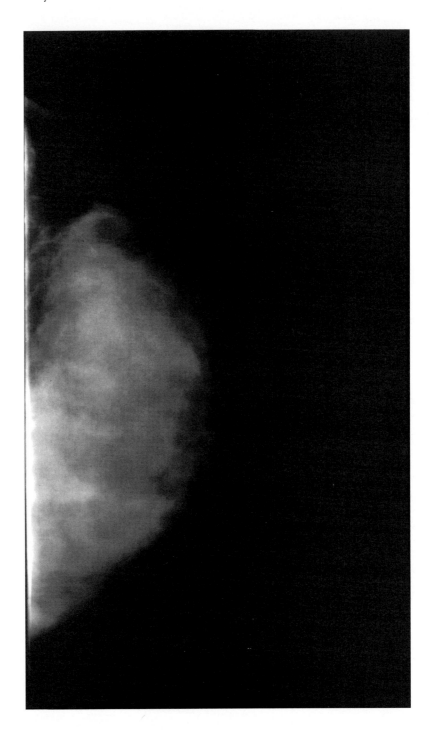

SOLUTION 2

The compression paddle is misaligned with the screen/film cassette so that the edge of the compression paddle is imaged on the film. The physicist's tests should have discovered this fault.

PROBLEM 3

Fine grid-like lines are present in the axillary portion of this mammogram, but they are perpendicular to the direction of true grid lines. What causes this pattern?

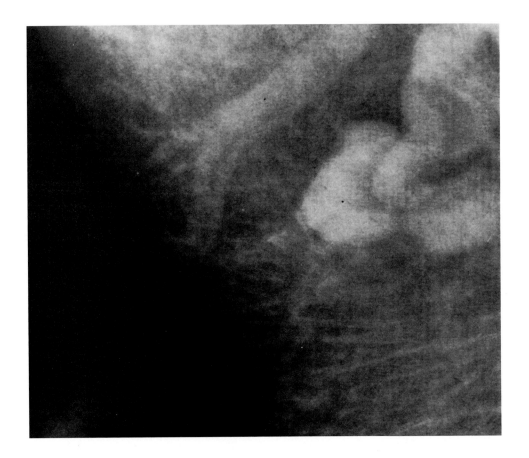

SOLUTION 3

Cloth adhesive tape (rather than plastic or fiber radiotranslucent tape) was placed on the cassette holder because it was abraded. The woven tape can be seen in fine detail because it is close to the screen/film combination.

PROBLEM 4

This is an image of the American College of Radiology mammography phantom. The insert is made of a uniform thickness of wax that has been embedded with masses, calcifications, and fibers. The background is supposed to be of uniform density except where these objects are located. What causes the light stripes running down the image? They are present in the same place on each phantom image.

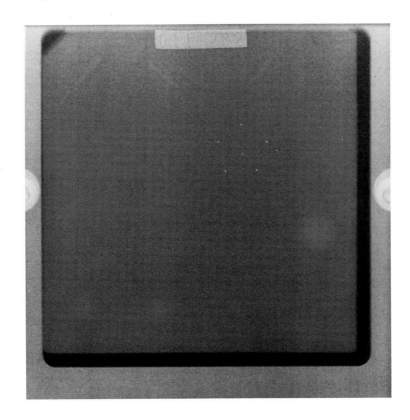

SOLUTION 4

All mammography units are supplied with a Mo and sometimes with a Rh filter to further shape the x-ray energy spectrum. Small variations in the thickness of this filter can cause these stripes. They will be in the same place on every image, unlike film processor roller marks that will vary in direction depending on how the film is fed into the processor.

QUESTIONS

1. Which requires more contrast, chest radiographs or mammograms?

2. What are the advantages and disadvantages of using a Rh anode instead of a Mo anode?

3. Why can't mammography focal spots used for non-magnified imaging be made smaller so that tiny calcifications can be seen more clearly?

4. If Rh anodes improve penetration, do breasts imaged with these anodes need to be compressed?

5. What factor is responsible for the greatest increase in dose to the patient: the screen/film combination, method of film processing, generator and x-ray tube output, anode/filter combination, extent of compression, or "retakes"?

6. Why are quality and dose more carefully regulated for mammograms than for chest x-rays?

ANSWERS

1. Mammograms require more contrast because the attenuation difference between glandular tissue and carcinoma is so small. As kVp increases, this difference all but disappears so that even using a film which has high contrast cannot reproduce an image of the carcinoma.

2. Because the photoelectric peaks are about 3 keV higher for Rh, the spectrum of energy emitted from a Rh anode is about 3 keV higher (23 keV) than that of a Mo anode spectrum. Because soft tissue contrast depends on the attenuation differences between glandular tissue and abnormal tissue, a difference that decreases with increasing kVp, contrast is reduced in mammograms obtained with a Rh anode. This loss of contrast is the major disadvantage. The advantages of using a Rh anode x-ray tube is that large and dense breasts can be penetrated by the higher energy spectrum more readily, leading to shortened exposure times and fewer motion artifacts. In addition, fewer low energy photons remain in the breast to contribute to the radiation dose.

3. The smaller the focal spot, the fewer electrons it can emit per second to travel to the anode and produce x-ray photons. Were the mA increased in a small cathode, the extra heat generated might destroy it. The low x-ray photon flux leads to a long exposure, since a certain number of photons per emission area is needed to darken the film sufficiently. If very high speed screen film combinations are used that require less photon flux, resolution will be poor due to screen blurring. Thus there is an interdependence between focal spot size, filament overheating, photon flux, patient motion, screen/film speed, and resolution.

4. Yes, because compression doesn't just flatten the breast to allow the low energy x-ray photons to penetrate it, it also equalizes the thickness of the breast, equalizing the range of tissue attenuation that must be displayed on the film. Without compression, we could not use high contrast film. In addition, compression spreads out the tissue so that it covers a greater area, decreasing the overlap of anatomic and pathologic structures and improving the depiction of abnormalities.

5. If several "retakes" are needed, the dose is doubled for each retake. However, some screen/film combinations require twice the dose of others, so they can also cause a significant increase in dose. Compressing the patient's breast to 4 cm instead of 5 cm can decrease the dose to the breast by almost half as well as decrease the time of the exposure, which helps prevent motion. Use of W or Rh anodes may decrease the dose by 40–50%, but this should be performed only for large or dense breasts. Film processing, the generator, and x-ray tube output affect dose by only about 20%.

6. A posteroanterior chest radiograph requires a skin exposure of only 15 mR, whereas the skin exposure for a mammogram is almost 1 R, about 60 times the exposure dose. Because of the differences in the energy spectrum used for the two modalities (25 vs. 110 kVp for chest radiographs), the internal dose is calculated differently so that although a chest radiograph

may deliver 10 mrad to the liver, mean glandular dose to the breast is about 150 mrad. Because the potential of mammography radiation to cause a malignancy decreases mammography's benefit-to-risk ratio, we must be careful that each mammogram is performed in such a way that a cancer, if present, is detected, justifying the minuscule risk of carcinogenesis from the radiation dose. Chest radiographs, being associated with much less risk and less challenge to image quality, may be regulated less carefully.

2

GETTING STARTED

Dedicated mammography units are now mandated for breast imaging. Comparison between the images made with a dedicated unit and those made with general purpose equipment illustrates why dedicated mammography units are required (Fig. 2.1). In addition to high quality x-ray equipment, proper positioning and film processing are essential. Although mammography units are relatively inexpensive compared with some other radiographic equipment, they can be used only for breast imaging. Dedicated mammography units may differ in price by as much as $60,000. Questions will arise about which options to purchase and where savings can be made without adverse effects on image quality.

There are many ways to reduce equipment costs. Some manufacturers lease equipment or offer used equipment with a warranty. If only screening examinations are to be performed, a microfocal spot, magnification stand, and special compression paddles are not required. A modest decrease in the capabilities of a less expensive unit, in comparison with a full-service unit, may be acceptable for a low volume mammography facility.

This chapter will discuss equipment tradeoffs and options for mammography units; quality control equipment needed by the radiologic technologist is also explained. Image receptors and processing equipment will be covered in subsequent chapters. Some concepts presented in this chapter are supplemented by material in later chapters. Some readers may wish to defer this chapter until after they have read more of the workbook. An excellent related publication by the American College of Radiology (ACR) (see Yaffe et al. under "Suggested Readings") should prove to be a useful guide for the reader.

PREVIOUSLY OWNED EQUIPMENT

The attempt to reduce initial capital expenditures by purchasing previously owned (used) mammography equipment that is older than 3 years is not recommended for several reasons: it precludes the benefits of ongoing design improvements, and x-ray tubes have a finite life and may cost as much as $24,000 to replace. If the used unit has been in storage more than a few months, the chance of tube failure is increased significantly. We also do not recommend purchasing used mammography equipment without specific guarantees from the manufacturer and then only if a competent medical physicist who specializes in mammography can first test the unit. However, if the manufacturer will agree to sell a 1-year warranty (parts and service) with the unit and defer payment until the unit passes both ACR accreditation testing and a thorough medical physicist's survey, then used equipment may fill the need for a start-up mammography facility. The physicist can judge the age of the x-ray tube by the half value layer of aluminum measurement and by the tube output. As a mammography tube ages, its filament thins, and atoms from the filament progressively coat the beryllium window, causing the half value layer to exceed 0.35 mm of aluminum at 26 kVp. In addition, longer exposures are needed to penetrate the metalized x-ray tube window so that < 8 mR/mAs may be measured at 26 kVp. Additionally, automatic exposure controls on older mammography units cannot produce the same optical density as those on newer units for varying thicknesses of breast tissue. If a used unit cannot produce images of 2-, 4-, and 6-cm thicknesses of acrylic within 0.3 optical density of each other, clinical images are unlikely to be satisfactorily exposed.

All cassette holders, grids, and compression paddles should be inspected for damage caused by wear and mishandling by the previous users. Reciprocating grids rather than fixed grids must be installed. Appropriate compression paddles and cassette holders must be available for 18×24 cm and 24×30 cm image receptors. Collimation should meet ACR recommendations, because excessive collimation will adversely affect film viewing conditions, allowing view box light to pass through unexposed areas of the film (Fig. 2.2).

NEW EQUIPMENT SPECIFICATIONS

Mammography equipment manufacturers now produce equipment that is generally compliant with ACR and Mammography Quality Standards Act (MQSA) regulations. However, if a new model that has not previously

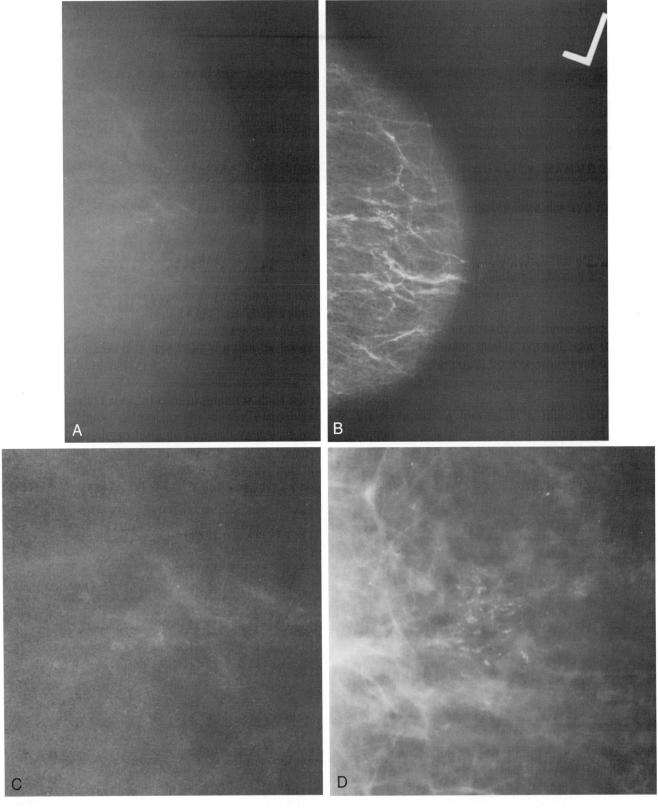

Figure 2.1. **A.** Image made with nondedicated radiographic equipment. **B.** Same breast imaged with a dedicated Mo anode unit. **C.** Detail of cluster of calcifications shown in **A. D.** Detail of the cluster of calcifications shown in **B.**

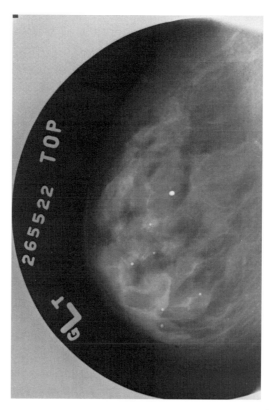

Figure 2.2. Many older mammography units collimate the breast to reduce scattered radiation. Unexposed film permits light from the view box to interfere with correct mammography viewing conditions.

been accredited is to be purchased, a determination should be made regarding whether all the basic recommended specifications have been met (see Yaffe et al. under "Suggested Readings"). If the unit is to be used for magnification, compression spot views, or biopsies, the following additional equipment is needed.

1. A magnification stand at one-third the source-to-image distance is required to provide magnification of 1.5–1.6, depending on breast thickness. Magnification requires a microfocal spot (0.1- to 0.15-mm nominal width).
2. Additional compression paddles for spot views (which may be combined with magnification) are needed.
3. A fenestrated (windowed) compression plate or hole plate (one with 1-cm-diameter holes spaced every 0.5 cm) is needed for localization, cyst aspiration, and fine-needle aspiration biopsy procedures (see Chapter 4).
4. An add-on stereotactic biopsy device may be useful if a sufficient number of procedures are anticipated.

ADDITIONAL MAMMOGRAPHY OPTIONS

Several improvements in mammography equipment have recently become available. A Rh filter is available for breasts that are difficult to penetrate. This filtration tends to reduce bremsstrahlung radiation by k-edge filtering much of the radiation above 23 keV and by reducing the Mo k-edge radiation centered at 20 keV. A more effective but more expensive option is found in equipment with dual anode tracks, allowing use of either W or Rh; when a Rh filter is deployed, the anode is better matched to the filter. In the case of a W anode, a much thicker Rh filter is needed (0.05 mm) than the Mo filter (0.03 mm). This reduces the available mA, but because the photons have higher energy (23 rather than 20 keV), exposures are shorter. High-volume facilities with multiple mammography units may wish to invest in a dual anode unit.

Some manufacturers have positioning aids on their units. One unit has built-in 18 × 24 and 24 × 30 cm grids, simplifying the changing of the image receptor size, and the height of the c-arm does not have to be adjusted to perform the mediolateral view after performing the craniocaudal view. Another unit allows compression to be completed by movement of the cassette holder, where the breast tissue is movable rather than fixed. Several units allow women to lean forward into the compression device so that breast tissue falls naturally away from the chest wall. These positioning aids require special training for the technologist. If equipment with these options is ordered, verify the length of time an applications specialist will be available to train the technologist at your facility and whether the specialist will return to your facility without charge if new technologists need to be trained.

Fixed grids are no longer recommended for mammography; some manufacturers have introduced innovative moving grids, including a honeycomb grid that provides two-dimensional rather than one-dimensional scatter cleanup.

Automatic exposure control systems are now more complex. Units with Rh filters and Rh or W anodes offer automatic kVp, anode, and filter selection as well as automatic mAs selection. Some of these programs are more reliable than others, and all must be checked carefully by a medical physicist during acceptance testing.

Automatic compression, i.e., compression which senses that the breast is sufficiently compressed for imaging, is also available and has been shown to be generally acceptable.

All these features add to equipment cost, require additional training of radiologic technologists, and warrant careful acceptance testing by a qualified medical physicist.

MEDICAL PHYSICIST SELECTION, COST, AND EQUIPMENT

Selecting a physicist to perform acceptance tests on your new equipment may be difficult in some geographic regions. Transportation and hotel costs as high as $500 may be required if a physicist who specializes in mammography is unavailable in your area. Most physicists charge from $90 to $150 per hour. Mammography acceptance testing may require from 3 to 8 hours, depending on the difficulties encountered and the skill and experience of the physicist. This time can be reduced by as much as 25% if a technologist is available to process radiographs during the tests. Preparation of a report may require another 1–2 hours. Some states offer lists of physicists who are registered with the state to check diagnostic x-ray equipment. Do not be reticent about asking the physicists for references concerning their experience with mammography equipment. Although MQSA requirements for the background and training of mammography physicists guarantee that they will have some familiarity with mammography, they may not be familiar with the particular equipment you have purchased. It is cost-effective to have the manufacturer's service engineer

present during acceptance testing so that deficiencies can be corrected and the machine retested.

One benefit of complete acceptance testing is that it provides a baseline for ongoing quality assurance checks and for troubleshooting in the event of equipment failure. Therefore, the tests should be fully documented, and all phantom images should be retained for comparison purposes.

NEGOTIATING A CONTRACT

The cost of acceptance testing of a mammography unit is borne by the imaging facility. However, the buyer may wish to stipulate in the equipment purchase contract that if the equipment fails to pass acceptance testing, subsequent visits by the physicist will be paid for by the manufacturer until the defect has been satisfactorily repaired. The buyer should also be aware that if he or she pays 90% of the equipment cost before it is tested, the supplier may "walk away" from a deficient unit if the cost of its repair is more than the remaining 10%. This is especially likely if the supplier is an agent, rather than an employee, of the manufacturer. Agents representing the manufacturers include in the purchase price the cost of installation and service. If they cannot recover the installation cost, they may be slow to correct problems, electing instead to challenge the physicist's results. A carefully written contract that stipulates that at least 20% of the payment is to be deferred until acceptance tests are satisfactory will save the buyer delays and unexpected expenses.

Once the unit is accepted, the ACR accreditation process can begin. This procedure will require that specified quality control procedures are followed for evaluating the processor and equipment. Processing and screen/film cassettes will be discussed in subsequent chapters. However, certain basic quality control equipment is required before the accreditation process commences.

(*a*) Processor testing can begin before the mammography unit has been delivered. Simulation of radiographic exposures can be achieved by running 30 light-exposed films per day; densitometric values can be plotted each morning to establish processor stability. A dedicated sensitometer designed for mammography film and a densitometer should be purchased for this quality control task.

(*b*) An ACR accreditation phantom should be ordered when the mammography unit is ordered. The physicist will make a control image of this phantom during acceptance testing. This control image can then be compared with subsequent images of the same phantom to ensure consistent imaging quality.

(*c*) Within the first 6 months of operation, several additional test devices will be needed:
- Bathroom scale (nondigital);
- Mammography screen film contact mesh;
- Fixer clearance test kit;
- A 2-cm-thick piece of 24×30 cm acrylic.

(*d*) Notebooks and quality assurance forms to record the quality assurance test results and other documentation required by MQSA should be organized in a convenient manner before an MQSA inspection.

SITE PREPARATION

Its low kVp output precludes mammography equipment from requiring the extensive room shielding needed for general purpose radiology equipment. Because laws are based on the maximum kVp that can be used in a room, be sure to stipulate that your mammography unit does not produce x-rays higher than 35 kVp. Radiation shielding can then be directed toward protection from scattered radiation. Gypsum wallboards 5/8-inch thick are recommended. A double thickness attenuates the beam to 0.000065 of its original value.

To protect patient privacy, the breast imaging and changing rooms should be isolated from the general radiographic rooms.

A mammography reading room should contain a shuttered, high intensity viewer designed specifically for mammography. The room should have no external windows, and ambient light from hallways, adjacent rooms, and x-ray view boxes should be minimized.

Suggested Readings

Bassett LW, Hendrick RE, Bassford TL, et al. Quality determinants of mammography. Clinical practice guideline no. 13. Rockville MD: Agency for Health Care Policy and Research, Public Health Service, Department of Health and Human Services, Oct 1994 (AHCPR publication 95-0632).

Chapter 5, "Responsibilities of the Mammography Facility," recommends particular attributes of mammography equipment and backs up these recommendations with published references. This pamphlet is an excellent source of references for all aspects of mammography. To order single copies of guideline products or to obtain further information on their availability, contact AHCPR Publications Clearinghouse, PO box 8547, Silver Spring MD 20907 (1-800-358-9295).

Strauss KJ, Rossi RP. Specification, acceptance testing and quality control of mammographic imaging equipment. In: Haus AG, Yaffe MJ, eds. Syllabus: a categorical course in physics. Technical aspects of breast imaging, 3rd ed. Radiological Society of North America 80th Annual Meeting, Nov 27–Dec 2, 1994.

This chapter goes into great detail concerning the performance parameters to be specified in a purchase order for a mammography unit. Tables are given that, if followed, should prevent lack of compliance or any misunderstandings between the vendor and buyer.

Yaffe MJ, Hendrick RE, Feig SA, Rothenberg LN, Och J, Gagne R. Recommended specifications for new mammography equipment: report of the ACR-CDC focus group on mammography equipment. Radiology 1995;197:19–26.

This publication describes all components needed for quality mammography, including the x-ray system, quality control equipment, mammography viewers, image receptors, and film processors. Each requirement includes a short explanation.

PROBLEM 1

The breast shown here was imaged with a 24 × 30 cm grid. Why is this film unsatisfactory?

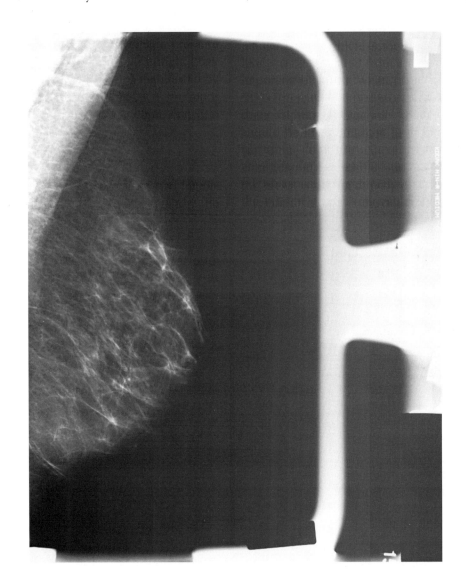

SOLUTION 1

The breast could easily fit on an 18 × 24 cm film. The 18 × 24 compression paddle was used instead of the 24 × 30 cm paddle so that the structure of the compression paddle inappropriately appears on the film. Each cassette holder has a matching compression paddle. Some manufacturers also supply 24 × 30 cm compression paddles with an additional 5-cm lip at the chest wall to push supramammary subcutaneous fat away from the film plane.

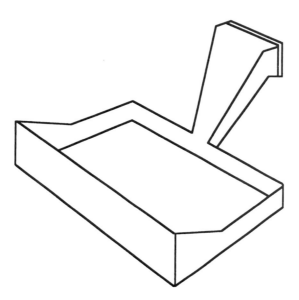

PROBLEM 2

These calcifications were imaged with four different focal spots. Can you rank them from sharpest to most blurred? What does your ranking imply regarding the focal spots used to image these calcifications?

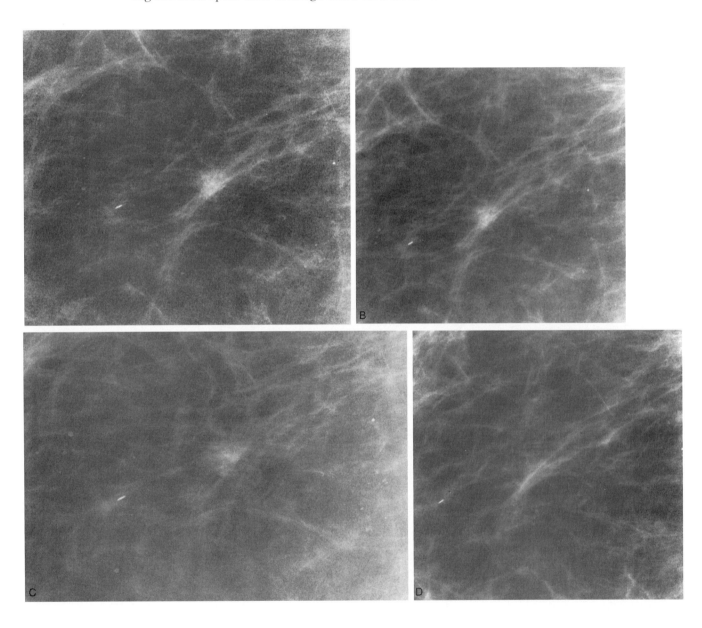

SOLUTION 2

Panels B and *C* were imaged with the same microfocal spot, but *panel* C is a magnified x-ray image, whereas *panel B* is a contact image. *Panel A* was imaged with a 0.3-mm focal spot, whereas the focal spot that imaged *panel D* was 0.42 mm wide.

PROBLEM 3

The image below contains a mass behind the nipple of this 6.5-cm-thick breast. Why does the detail of the mass lack clarity, even though a Mo anode, Mo filter technique was used?

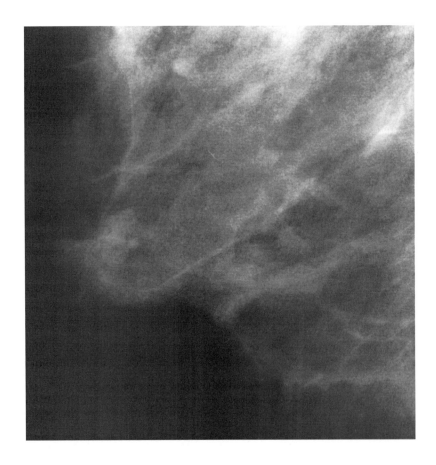

SOLUTION 3

A fixed grid was employed in the previous image. When a reciprocating grid is used, the mass is clearly visible.

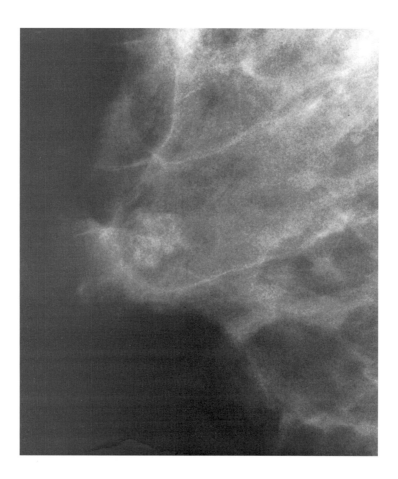

PROBLEM 4

The image below is limited in diagnostic content because glandular tissue is not penetrated. A reciprocating grid and high contrast film have been used. The automatic exposure control selected 29 kVp and 200 mAs as the technique. What would you suggest?

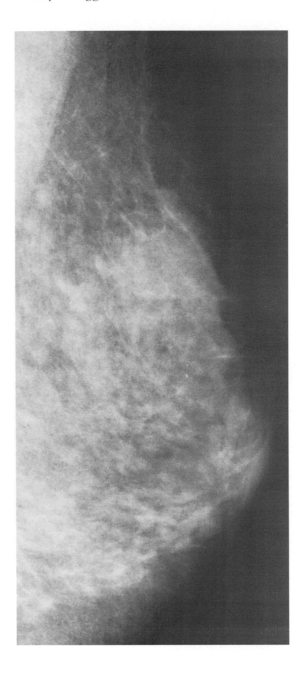

SOLUTION 4

Image the breast with a W anode or Rh anode and Rh filter at 26 or 27 kVp. This image represents the same breast imaged with a Rh anode and Rh filtration.

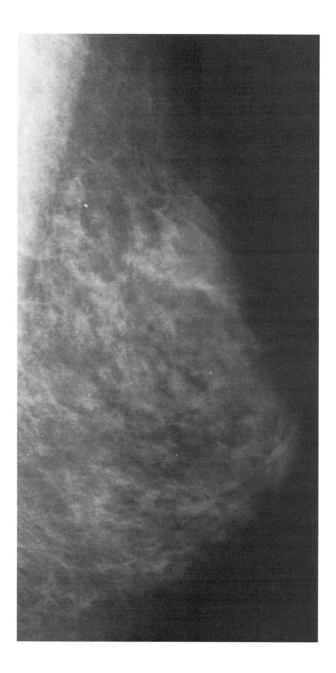

QUESTIONS

1. A manufacturer replaces the x-ray tube on your old mammography unit. The service engineer images your ACR mammography accreditation phantom, and 10 objects can be seen in it. Should the unit be tested by a medical physicist?

2. The automatic exposure control produces films with the same optical density for 2-, 4-, and 6-cm-thick pieces of acrylic so long as kVp can vary with increasing slab thickness. However, if only 26 kVp is used when imaging these pieces of acrylic, optical density varies from 1.8 to 0.8. Is this satisfactory (be-cause you would probably raise the kVp for a 6-cm breast anyway)?

3. If 75% of the patients in your practice are older than 60, should you still consider purchasing a mammography unit with Rh filtration?

4. An imaging center already has three sensitometers. For daily processor quality control, can the mammography technologist borrow whichever one is not being used?

5. Your practice is located in a region where most women have large breasts and require a 24 × 30 cm image receptor. Can you use the large image receptor with small cassettes for the few women with smaller breasts who come to your facility?

ANSWERS

1. Yes. The x-ray tube must meet ACR and MQSA resolution requirements. In addition, other tests by the physicist are affected by the x-ray tube change, such as those of kVp, half value layer, mean glandular dose, automatic exposure control, and collimation. (Expect to pay the physicist about 75% of the cost of a yearly survey.)

2. The ACR requires that the automatic exposure control maintain film optical density within ± 0.3 optical density of the average optical density over all the slab thicknesses. It does not require that all exposures be obtained at the same kVp but at clinically relevant kVp values.

3. Yes, because many women older than 60 receive estrogenic hormonal therapy that tends to preserve or increase glandular tissue. Furthermore, women with large breasts of > 6 cm in compressed thickness will benefit from the reduced dose offered by Rh filtration.

4. The same sensitometer must be used each day for mammography sensitometry. If the imaging center can assign one of the three sensitometers to mammography, and if the sensitometry light spectrum and optical wedge values are appropriate for mammography film, then the facility does not need to purchase a new sensitometer.

5. Even if the 24 × 30 cm cassette holder has an insert to hold the 18 × 24 cm image receptor in place, this will not be satisfactory. The large grid will not fit into the axilla of small patients on the mediolateral oblique view if the small cassette is centered in the large grid holder.

3

EVALUATION OF CLINICAL IMAGES

Clinical images should be evaluated for technical quality by both the radiologic technologist performing the examination and the radiologist interpreting the examination as an ongoing quality control activity. Learning to recognize deficiencies in clinical images and their possible causes will allow the mammography team to correct problems efficiently. Occasionally, determining the exact source of a clinical image problem will require exposure of a phantom image and consultation with the medical physicist.

An external review of clinical images is now mandated by the Mammography Quality Standards Act of 1992. This external review must be performed at least every 3 years by specially trained qualified interpreting physicians under the auspices of an accrediting body approved by the Food and Drug Administration. For each mammography unit, the facility submits bilateral screening examinations of a woman with fatty breasts and of a woman with dense breasts. These two types of breast composition pose different imaging challenges. Owing to variations in the cooperation and body habitus of the women being examined, it is not possible to attain ideal breast positioning and compression in all cases. Therefore, facilities are requested to submit what they consider to be good representative images.

The process of evaluation of clinical images involves an assessment of each of the following determinants of image quality: positioning, compression, contrast, exposure, noise, sharpness, artifacts, collimation, and labeling. A recent evaluation of data from the American College of Radiology Mammography Accreditation Program revealed that the most frequent problems occurred with breast positioning. Therefore, this chapter includes an extensive section on the assessment of breast positioning through the evaluation of clinical images. Compression, exposure, and sharpness accounted for the next greatest numbers of deficiencies in clinical images.

POSITIONING

Breast positioning has continued to improve over the years so that mammograms from only a few years ago might not be acceptable by the most recent criteria. Improvements in positioning can be attributed to advances in dedicated mammography equipment, a better understanding of the anatomy of the breast and its mobility, and required educational programs for radiologic technologists. The mediolateral oblique (MLO) and the craniocaudal (CC) views are the standard views for all screening and diagnostic examinations. The major goal in positioning a patient for a screening examination is to show all breast tissue on this combined two-view examination.

Mediolateral Oblique View

The MLO view (Fig. 3.1) offers the best opportunity to show all breast tissue in one image. Because the breast lies primarily on the pectoralis major muscle, a generous amount of the muscle should be included in the image. This assures that as much breast tissue as possible is included and as many cancers as possible are depicted (Fig. 3.2). More muscle can be included if the C-arm is rotated so that the Bucky (also called cassette holder or positioning table) is parallel to the plane of the pectoralis muscle (Fig. 3.1A). The mobile lateral border of the breast is moved as far toward the fixed medial border as possible before placing the breast on the cassette holder. The muscle should be as relaxed as possible, evidenced by a generous amount of muscle on the image and a triangular shape with a convex border anteriorly (Fig. 3.1B).

It is also desirable to see fat posterior to all fibroglandular tissue. If the fibroglandular tissue extends all the way to the posterior edge of the film, it must be assumed that some fibroglandular tissue is excluded from the image.

The breast should be positioned on the imaging receptor to allow visualization of as much of the breast and axilla as possible (Fig. 3.1A). If the breast is positioned too high or too low on the Bucky, the axilla or the inferior aspect of the breast can be "cut off" the image.

Proper positioning methods are required during the initiation and application of breast compression for the MLO. The breast will fall or "sag" if it is not held up by

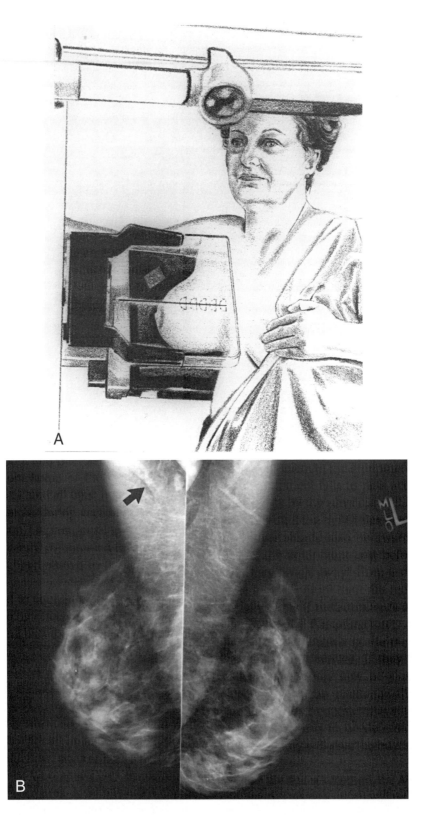

Figure 3.1.   MLO view. **A.** Final positioning for MLO view. C-arm of mammography unit has been rotated until cassette holder is parallel to the pectoral muscle. Breast is positioned on the cassette holder so that as much breast as possible will be seen. Line on plastic compression plate indicates plane of automatic exposure device. **B.** Bilateral MLO views. A generous amount of pectoral muscle has been included in the images. Muscle is triangular with slight anterior convexity. Note skin fold (*arrow*) in the axilla, a common finding that does not interfere with image interpretation.

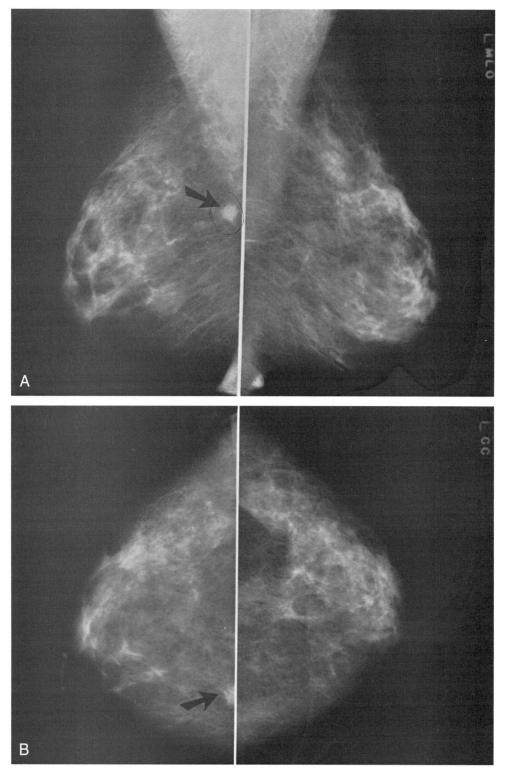

Figure 3.2. Right and left MLO (**A**) and right and left CC (**B**) views reveal a cancer (*arrows*) deep in the medial aspect of the breast. This small nonpalpable cancer would have been missed if a generous amount of pectoral muscle were not included in the MLO and if the CC had not been performed properly.

the technologist's hand until there is adequate pressure by the compression device to maintain an upright position of the breast. Sagging of the breast is manifested by a low position of the nipple on the image, superimposition of subareolar tissues, and a prominent skin fold near the inframammary fold (Fig. 3.3).

Craniocaudal View

The CC (Fig. 3.4) complements the MLO in two important ways. First, the CC can more effectively show the medial tissue, which is the portion of the breast most likely to be excluded from an MLO (Fig. 3.4B). Thus, an important objective when positioning the breast for the CC is to include all posteromedial tissue. This should be done without exaggerated positioning, and the nipple should be in the midline in the image. Second, the CC can often depict structures more clearly because more compression is possible, and motion is unlikely because the breast is resting directly on the cassette holder. Since the inferior tissue is movable and the superior tissue is

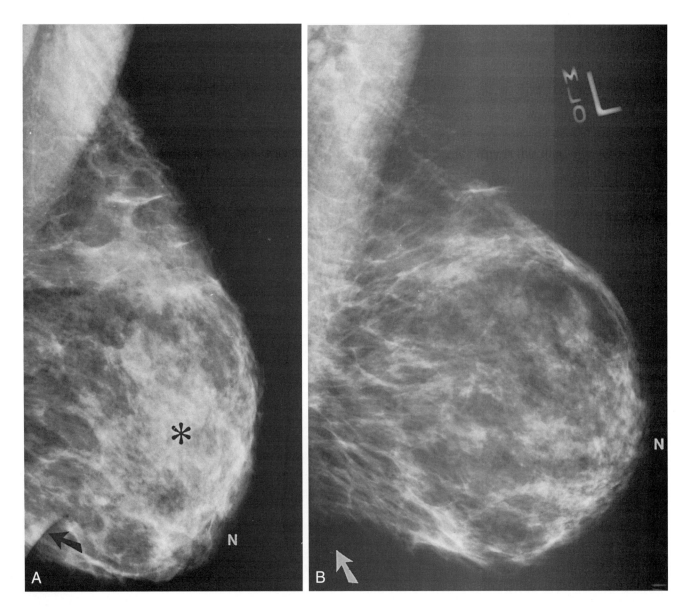

Figure 3.3. Sagging breast versus same breast properly positioned. **A.** In the sagging breast, the nipple (N) is located very low in the image, subareolar fibroglandular tissue (*asterisk*) is not well separated, and there is a prominent skin fold (*arrow*) at the posteroinferior aspect of the breast. **B.** Same breast properly positioned. Nipple is higher in the image, the subareolar tissues are well separated, and the inframammary fold (*arrow*) is open. Note that more pectoral muscle is shown.

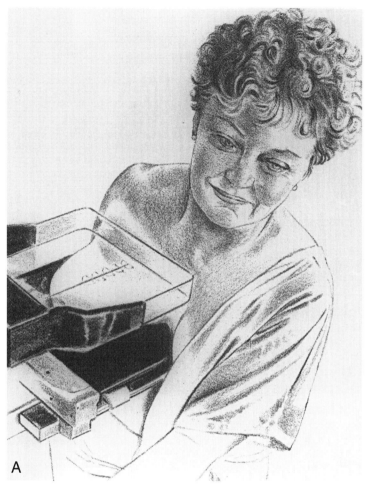

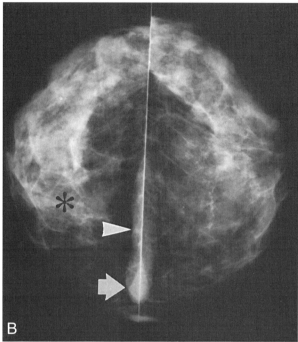

Figure 3.4. CC view. **A.** Final positioning for CC view. Technologist's hand has been used to elevate the breast so that the patient's shoulder is not far from the compression device. The nipple is positioned in the midline of the image receptor, without exaggeration to the medial or lateral side. The contralateral breast is draped over the side of the cassette holder rather than placed behind it. **B.** Bilateral CC views. Lateral aspect of the breast is at the top of the images. The pectoral muscle (*arrowhead*) is seen along the posteromedial aspect of the image. *Arrow,* accessory muscle called the sternalis muscle. All medial fibroglandular tissue (*asterisk*) has been imaged.

fixed, the radiologic technologist can improve the amount of tissue imaged by placing the hand under the inframammary fold and lifting the breast as high as possible before placing the breast on the Bucky. Other positioning tips that experienced technologists report for increasing the amount of medial tissue shown include standing on the medial side of the breast being positioned and draping the contralateral breast over the edge of the Bucky rather than placing it behind the Bucky. Although the goal is to include all medial tissue, this should be done without exaggerating CC positioning, which would result in unnecessary exclusion of lateral tissue (Fig. 3.5). The radiologic technologist can pull additional lateral tissue onto the image once the medial tissue is adequately positioned.

Image Analysis

There are several reliable image criteria to determine whether the breasts were properly positioned for the MLO and CC views. For the MLO view, the amount of pectoral muscle and the shape of the muscle on the image are important (Fig. 3.6). Whenever possible the muscle should extend to the posterior nipple line or below. The location of the nipple and the presence of an open inframammary fold are additional criteria. Each criterion can be achieved in approximately 85% of patients.

For the CC view the criteria are different (Fig. 3.6*B*). If the pectoral muscle is visualized in the posterior aspect of the image we can assume that there is adequate visualization of posterior tissue. However, the pectoral muscle is only visualized in about 30% of properly per-

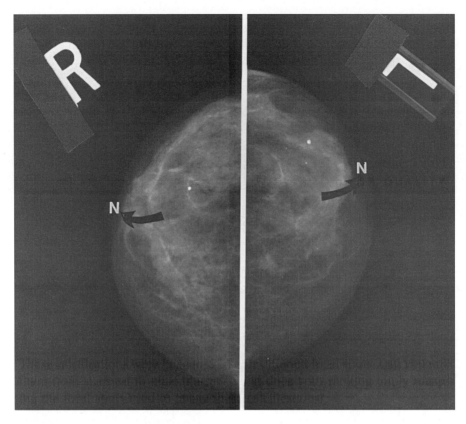

Figure 3.5. Exaggerated positioning of right and left CC views. All medial tissue has been imaged, but the patient was rotated laterally (*arrows*) to accomplish this, as evidenced by the lateral position of the nipples (N), especially the left nipple. This results in unnecessary exclusion of lateral tissue.

formed CC views. If the pectoral muscle is *not* seen, the length of a line drawn directly posterior to the nipple and extending to the posterior edge of the film (posterior nipple line) is the most reliable indicator of whether enough posterior tissue is included. A good general rule is that the length of the posterior nipple line on the CC should be within 1 cm of its length on the properly performed MLO of the same breast. On the CC, the posterior nipple line is drawn directly posterior from the nipple to the edge of the film. On the MLO the posterior nipple line is drawn at an angle of approximately 45° from the nipple to the pectoral muscle or the edge of the film (Fig. 3.6*A*). For the CC view the nipple should be in the midline position, and all medial fibroglandular tissue should be visible.

Additional Positioning Deficiencies

Skin folds over the surface of the breast should be avoided (Fig. 3.7). For the MLO view, the breast should be placed on the image receptor in such a manner that the axilla or inferior breast tissue is not excluded. Some radiologic technologists have been taught to always place the nipple at the center of the image on the MLO, at the level of the automatic exposure control device. This is often not the correct location for the nipple because it may place the breast too high on the image receptor, resulting in exclusion of axillary tissue. Likewise, placing the breast too low on the image will result in cut-off of inferior breast tissue.

Today, both 18 × 24 cm and 24 × 30 cm image receptors should be available for each mammography unit. If the image receptor is too small for the breast, a portion of either the axilla or inferior breast tissue will be excluded. If the image receptor is too large, the interposition of other body parts between the cassette and the breast may prevent adequate breast compression (Fig. 3.8).

COMPRESSION

Adequate breast compression is essential for high quality mammography. Compression decreases breast thickness, which reduces radiation dose, scattered ra-

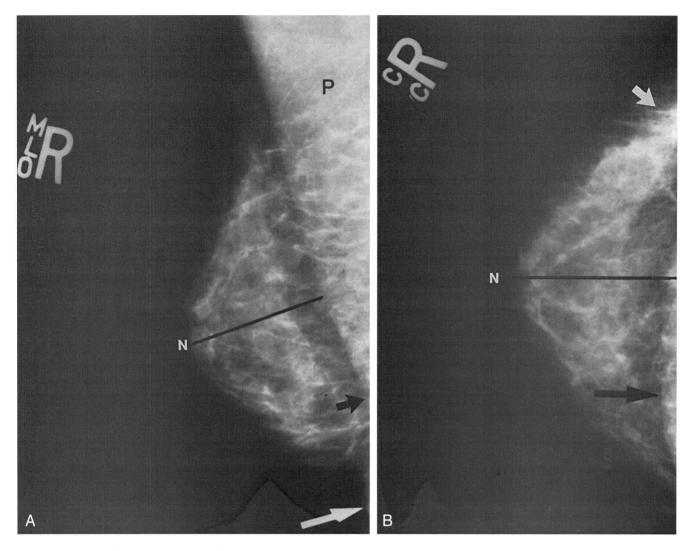

Figure 3.6. Positioning criteria for MLO and CC views. **A.** Properly positioned MLO view. Amount of pectoral muscle (P) should be generous, and insertion of the muscle (*black arrow*) should be at or below the posterior nipple line. Nipple (N) should be high in the image, and the inframammary fold (*white arrow*) should be open. **B.** Properly positioned CC view. Pectoral muscle (*black arrow*) at the posterior aspect of the breast confirms inclusion of deep posterior breast tissue. If the pectoral muscle is not present, the posterior nipple line is used to document adequate imaging of posterior tissue. Posterior nipple line on the CC should measure within 1 cm of its length on the MLO. Nipple should be in the midline, and all posteromedial fibroglandular tissue should be visualized.

diation, and geometric unsharpness. Furthermore, compression makes the thickness of the breast more uniform so that film optical densities are more likely to correspond to subtle attenuation differences rather than differences in tissue thickness. Uniform thickness also makes it possible to show all of the breast adequately on one image. Compression also eliminates motion unsharpness.

To be effective, the compression device should match the size of the image receptor and remain parallel to the image receptor during the application of compression. The posterior edge of the compression device should be straight, not curved. To ensure sustained compression of the thicker posterior tissues, the angle between the posterior lip and inferior surface of the compression device should be approximately 90° and not gently curved. The posterior surface of the compression device should be high enough, usually 3–4 cm, to prevent chest wall structures from being superimposed on the image of the breast.

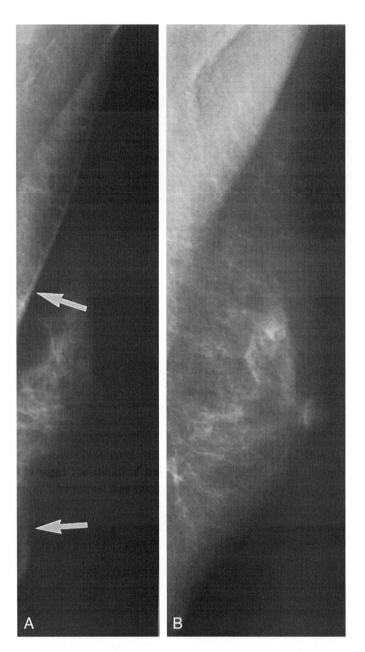

Figure 3.7. Skin folds. Because of the small size of the woman's breast it was difficult for the radiologic technologist to use the hand to hold the breast up and out while initiating compression for the MLO view. **A.** The result was large skin folds (*arrows*) superimposed on the image of the breast. **B.** Same breast with excellent compression and no skin folds. This was achieved by using a rubber kitchen spatula, in place of the technologist's hand, to hold up the breast during application of compression.

Experienced radiologic technologists achieve better compression by using the following techniques: (*a*) before applying compression they advise the woman of its importance and the benefits of relaxation; (*b*) they inform the woman before compression is initiated; (*c*) they apply the compression in gradations, with input from the woman regarding whether she can tolerate more; and (*d*) they increase the compression until the skin of the breast is taut but not painful.

Image Analysis. Inadequate compression is manifested by overlapping of breast structures (Figs. 3.3*A*, 3.8, and 3.9), nonuniform tissue exposure (Figs. 3.9*A* and 3.10), and motion unsharpness (Figs. 3.8, 3.9*A*, and 3.10). Motion caused by inadequate compression is more commonly seen on the MLO than the CC because the weight of the breast is completely supported by the Bucky on the CC view.

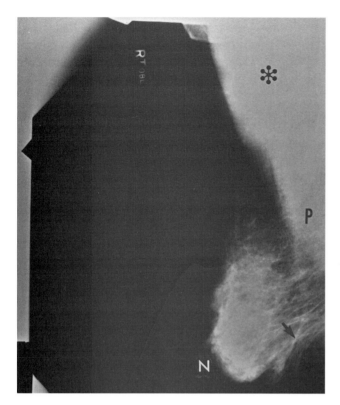

Figure 3.8. MLO performed on wrong size image receptor. A woman with small breasts was imaged on the larger (24 × 30 cm) image receptor. Adequate compression was prevented by the interposition of the shoulder structures (*asterisk*) above the pectoral muscle (P), which is underexposed. Evidence of inadequate compression include the low position of the nipple (N), poor separation and underexposure of fibroglandular tissue posterior to the nipple, and blurring of linear structures (*arrow*) in the inferior aspect of the breast caused by motion unsharpness.

CONTRAST

We can define radiographic contrast as the degree of variation in optical densities in different areas of the film. Contrast allows perception of attenuation differences in the breast tissues. The contrast in mammography image receptor systems has continued to improve (Fig. 3.11). In addition to the type of film that is used, radiographic contrast is also affected by subject contrast (radiation quality, kVp), exposure, film processing, and scatter reduction (compression, grids).

To achieve high contrast, kVp settings in the range of 25–27 are used with combinations of targets and filters developed especially for mammography. Underexposure also contributes to low contrast in mammograms (Fig. 3.12).

Film processing is one of the most important factors contributing to radiographic contrast. Film should be de-

veloped according to the manufacturer's specifications, and chemicals should be replenished as is appropriate for the volume of films that are processed. Longer processing times increase image contrast, but extended processing also increases the noise in the image because lower x-ray exposures are utilized and the improved contrast makes the noise more apparent. Processor temperature is also crucial, and the processor thermometer should be checked regularly for accuracy.

Image Analysis. There should be marked differences in the optical density of regions composed of fibroglandular tissue versus those composed of fat. Fibroglandular tissue should be light gray to white and regions of fat dark gray to black on the image (Fig. 3.12B). High contrast is desirable, but if the contrast is too high it may be impossible to see both thick and thin parts of the breast on the same image. Thus, a balance must be reached between contrast and latitude when selecting the type of film for mammography and the technical factors that are used.

EXPOSURE

X-ray exposure results in film blackening or increased optical density. Film exposure is proportional to the product of milliamperes of x-ray tube current and time of exposure. In general, mAs has its greatest effect on exposure, whereas kVp has its greatest effect on contrast.

The high contrast films and low kVp techniques used in mammography result in small exposure latitude. In other words, when using high contrast films, small kVp or mAs differences will result in relatively large variations in optical density. Therefore, kVp and mAs must be selected carefully, and automated exposure control performance must be precise over the range of kVp, breast thicknesses, and density values encountered in clinical practice. An experienced radiologic technologist can usually identify inadequate exposures based on the length of time of the audible exposure relative to the thickness of the breast.

Currently, underexposure is a more frequent problem than is overexposure. Underexposure is manifested by the inability to see details within dense fibroglandular tissue and failure to achieve adequate film blackening in low tissue density regions, e.g., fat and subcutaneous tissues (Fig. 3.12). Because lesions can be obscured within underexposed fibroglandular tissue, underexposure can result in false-negative examinations. It should also be emphasized that underexposure is an unrecoverable er-

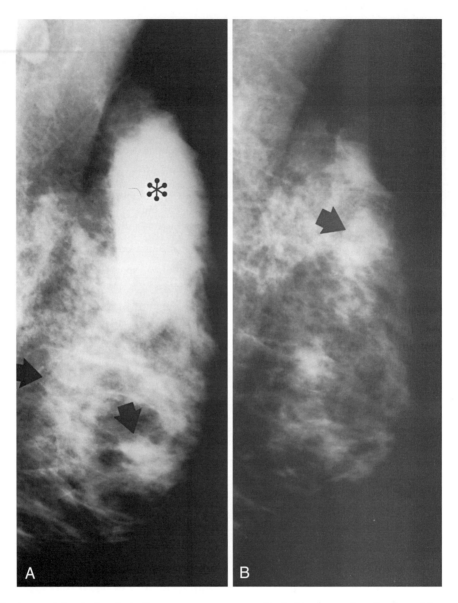

Figure 3.9. A patient complained of pain in the upper aspect of her left breast. **A.** Initial mammogram showed inadequate compression. A large area of poorly compressed fibroglandular tissue (*asterisk*) was underexposed and showed no structural details; other areas showed motion unsharpness, manifested by poor visualization of the margins of structures (*arrows*). **B.** Improved compression of the breast resulted in more uniform exposure and less blurring of structures. A circumscribed mass (*arrow*) was identified in the upper aspect of the breast, and this proved to be a cyst at ultrasonography.

ror that requires repeat imaging. However, overexposure is often a "recoverable" error in that it can be compensated for by using a high intensity view box light with masking of extraneous light or by "hot lighting" overexposed areas of the film with a bright light.

Image Analysis. Mammographic exposure should be evaluated under proper viewing conditions. The proper viewing conditions for mammography are addressed in the 1994 American College of Radiology Mammography

Quality Control manuals and include adequate view box luminance, low ambient room light (illuminance) to minimize light reflected off the surface of the film, and masking of films to prevent extraneous view box light that has not passed through the exposed areas of the film from reaching the eye. Appropriate viewing conditions for mammography can be achieved with dedicated mammography viewing equipment, but even these dedicated viewers need to be monitored for maintenance of adequate luminance. The view box surfaces should be

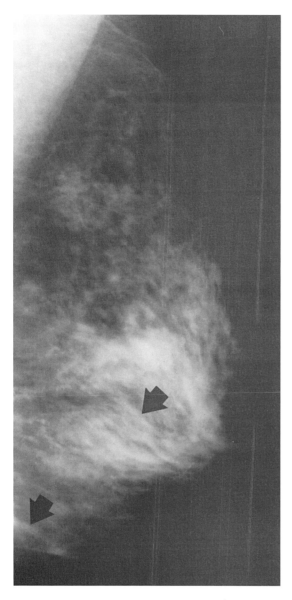

Figure 3.10. Inadequate compression and motion unsharpness. There is nonuniform exposure of the fibroglandular tissue and blurring of the linear structures (*arrows*) in the lower half of the breast.

cleaned once a week with the type of cleaner recommended by the manufacturer.

When the breasts are properly exposed and compressed the details within areas of dense fibroglandular tissue should be visible on the image. When the breast is adequately exposed it may be difficult to see details in the skin and subcutaneous tissues unless all extraneous view box light has been eliminated by masking around the edges of the films. On the MLO projection, the pectoralis muscle should be exposed sufficiently to show underlying tissue details (Fig. 3.1*B*). If the muscle

is underexposed (Fig. 3.8) it will not be possible to see breast tissue extending into the axillary region.

Overexposure is a less frequent problem in mammograms. It can result in loss of the visibility of structural details in the thin or fatty parts of the breast because of excessive blackening of the film.

NOISE

Noise, or radiographic mottle, compromises the ability to discern small details, e.g., calcifications in the breast. Radiographic mottle seen in mammograms is a composite of film grain, screen mottle, and quantum mottle. Quantum mottle, the most significant source of noise in mammography films, is due to a statistical fluctuation in the number of x-ray photons absorbed at individual locations in the intensifying screen. The fewer the number of x-ray photons that are used to make the image, or the lower the breast x-ray dose, the greater the amount of quantum mottle that will be observed in the image. Thus, film-screen systems that are faster, films that are underexposed, and extended processing all increase the noise in the image. Because noise can prevent the depiction of malignant calcifications or result in the illusion of tiny calcifications that are not there, a balance must be reached between low x-ray breast dose and acceptable image quality. For this reason, many faster film-screen combinations are being replaced by slower systems that require slightly greater x-ray dosage.

Image Analysis. An example of an unacceptably noisy image is shown under "Problem 2" in Chapter 6. Noise can be recognized as an irregular mottled appearance on the image resulting in an uneven texture. It is identified by looking carefully through a magnifying lens at areas with uniform density, e.g., an area of radiodense fibroglandular tissue. If mottle is pronounced, there may appear to be numerous faint "calcifications" throughout. Ironically, noise is more likely to be pronounced in high contrast films, because high contrast makes the mottle more visible.

SHARPNESS

Sharpness is the ability of the mammography system to define an edge. Unsharpness is often referred to as "blur." Types of unsharpness that occur in mammography include geometric, motion (Figs. 3.9*A* and 3.10), parallax and screen unsharpness, and blurring caused by poor film-screen contact (Fig. 3.13).

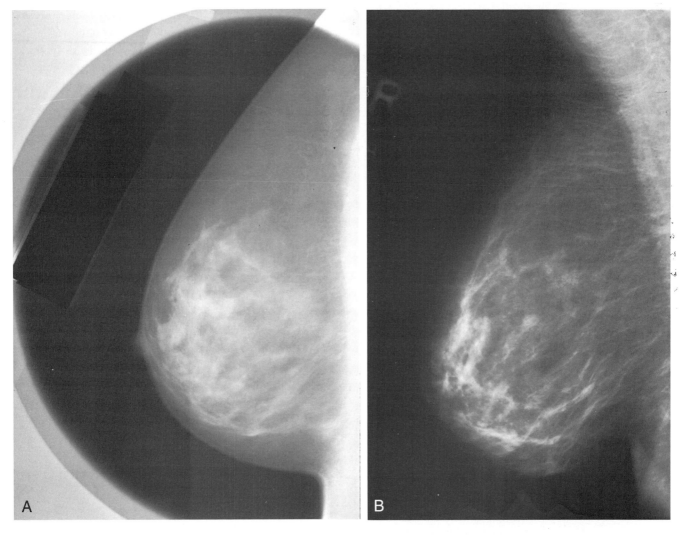

Figure 3.11. Improvements in radiographic contrast are demonstrated in mammograms of the same patient performed in 1975 (**A**) and 1992 (**B**).

An increase in focal spot size, a longer object-to-film distance, or a shorter source-to-image distance increases geometric unsharpness. Over the last decade, the focal spot sizes of dedicated mammography units have been reduced for both contact and magnification mammography. The source-to-image distance should be at least 55 cm for contact mammography and 60 cm for magnification mammography.

Parallax unsharpness refers to the blurring observed with the use of double-emulsion films. The image captured on each side of a double-emulsion film is separated by the width of the film base so that details will be slightly offset, resulting in some blurring of fine details. Because of the increased blur, double-emulsion films have not gained wide acceptance despite the lower radiation dose and longer tube life that they provide.

Screen unsharpness results from light diffusion. A single x-ray absorbed in the screen is converted to a large number of visible light photons, and the spread of these photons from the point of x-ray interaction in the screen to where they are absorbed by the film creates blurring of fine details. Faster screens, which are usually thicker, yield greater photon spread and increased screen unsharpness.

Any loss of intimate contact between the screen and the film results in the further spread of light from the screen before it reaches the film. Poor film-screen contact can result from poorly designed or damaged cassettes, improper placement of film in the cassette, dirt lying between the film and the screen (Fig. 3.13), or air trapped between the film and the screen at the time the film is loaded. It may take up to 15 minutes to achieve

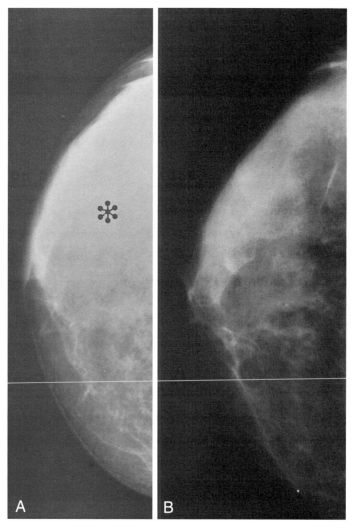

Figure 3.12. Underexposed (**A**) and properly exposed (**B**) mammograms. Underexposed image fails to show tissue details within dense fibroglandular tissue (*asterisk*) in the lateral aspect of the breast. Properly exposed mammogram shows more tissue details in the dense area and also improved contrast (greater differences in optical density between radiodense fibroglandular and radiolucent fatty tissue).

complete elimination of air after the cassette is loaded. Thus, the radiologic technologist should wait at least 15 minutes after loading cassettes before exposing them.

Image Analysis. Unsharpness is manifested by blurring of the edges of fine linear structures, tissue borders, and calcifications (Figs. 3.8, 3.9A, 3.10, and 3.13). A magnifying lens may be needed to perceive more subtle image blurring.

ARTIFACTS

An artifact can be defined as any density variation on the image that does not reflect true attenuation differences in the breast. Artifacts can reflect problems in darkroom cleanliness, film handling, screen maintenance, pro-cessing, or x-ray equipment. Objects or substances on the surface of the breast at the time of the exposure can also result in artifacts on the image.

The presence of multiple artifacts on images suggests problems in quality control at a facility. Many artifacts can be avoided by careful attention to darkroom conditions, including general cleanliness and regular mopping of the floors. Care in handling of films will avoid many artifacts. Regularly scheduled processor maintenance, re-plenishment of chemicals, cleaning of rollers, and daily quality assurance activities are essential.

Image Analysis. To identify artifacts, images should be inspected with a magnifying lens. Commonly encoun-

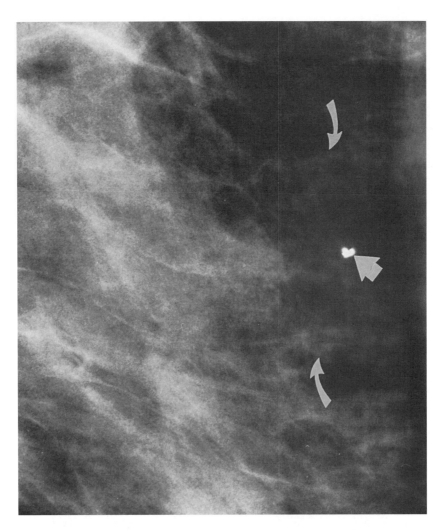

Figure 3.13. Unsharpness caused by poor film-screen contact. Close-up from area near the chest wall shows blurring of linear structures (*curved arrows*) caused by a piece of dirt (*broad arrow*) lying between film and screen.

tered artifacts include dust or lint, dirt (Fig. 3.13), scratches, fingerprints (Fig. 3.14), and fog. Many of these are demonstrated in other chapters in this workbook.

The film processor is the source of various artifacts, including roller marks, loader marks, and chemical residues. Artifacts related to the dedicated mammography unit include grid lines and improperly aligned equipment components that are superimposed on the image. For example, improper size, alignment, or design of the compression device can result in superimposition of the posterior lip over the posterior aspect of the image of the breast.

Various artifacts are due to substances or objects on the surface of the breast. Deodorant is one of the most commonly encountered of this type of artifact (Fig. 3.15). For this reason, many facilities ask women to delay the application of deodorants until their examination is completed. Body parts other than the breast can also be superimposed over the image of the breast. These include the patient's hair (Fig. 3.16) and the hand used to displace the contralateral breast from the area of the image (Fig. 3.17).

COLLIMATION

Collimating closely to the surface of the breast is discouraged because it can preclude effective masking of images at the view box (Figs. 3.11*A* and 3.18). The x-ray beam should be collimated to the edges of the image receptor, except posteriorly where the x-ray field should extend at least to the edge but may extend slightly beyond the edge of the image receptor. The latter allowance is to ensure that posterior breast tissue is not excluded from the image.

Image Analysis. Excessive collimation often results in excluding part of the breast from the image (Fig. 3.18). Round and curved collimators should not be used be-

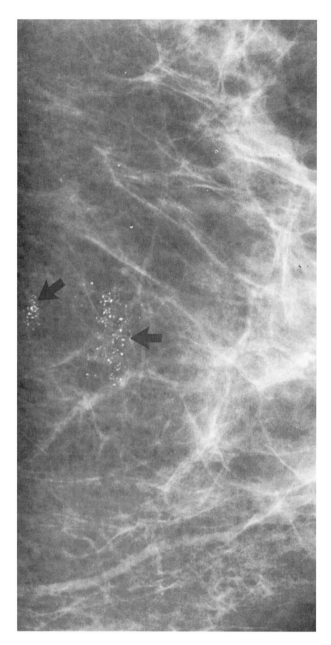

Figure 3.14. Close-up of mammogram reveals fingerprints (*arrows*) left on film during film loading that resulted in artifacts that simulated suspicious calcifications.

cause they prevent effective masking of the films at the view box. Ideally, the four sides of the collimator should each be straight and visualized slightly within the edges of the film, except posteriorly where the collimation should not be visible.

STANDARDIZED LABELING

Radiologists are frequently called on to review mammograms from other facilities. The dissemination of standardized labeling practices is intended to improve the quality of film labeling; eliminate confusion about view, laterality, and orientation of films; and to expedite the evaluation of films used for comparison or consultation. In 1993, a review of mammograms from facilities nationwide that were submitted to the American College of Radiology Mammography Accreditation Program for clinical image evaluation revealed a wide range of labeling practices, even among facilities in the same communities. Many mammograms did not contain enough information to adequately identify the facility or the examinee. Eccentric methods for designation of view and laterality were found to be confusing and could potentially lead to serious biopsy or treatment errors.

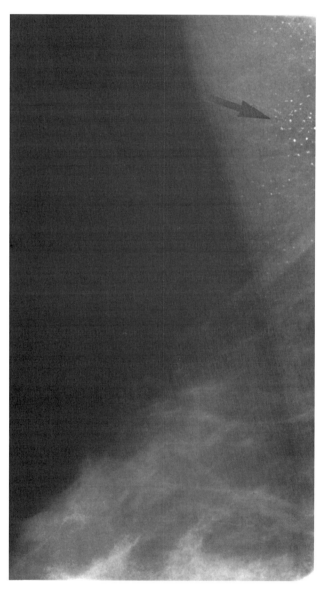

Figure 3.15. Close-up from MLO mammogram reveals deodorant residue (*arrows*) that simulates punctate calcifications in the axilla.

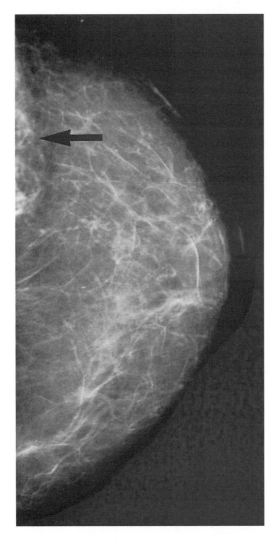

Figure 3.16. Patient's hair (*arrow*) is superimposed over posterior aspect of image.

It is strongly recommended that a "flash" type of identification label be used to ensure that the information will be permanent and that it can be transferred during film copying.

Optional labeling includes use of a paper date sticker that can be read with overhead light, a record of the film's technical factors (e.g., kVp, mAs, estimated breast compression), and the number (Roman numeral) of the dedicated mammography unit that was used.

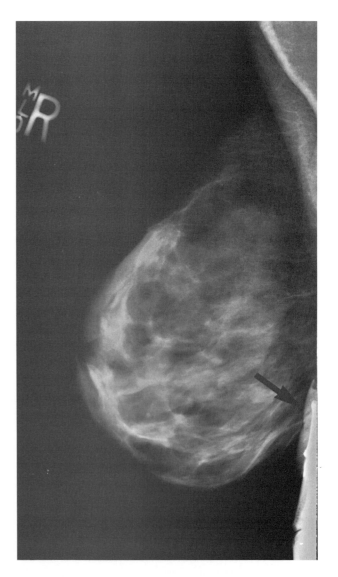

Figure 3.17. Patient's finger (*arrow*) from the hand displacing the contralateral breast is superimposed on posteroinferior aspect of this MLO.

Image Analysis. Required (essential) items include an identification label, laterality and view (Table 3.1), cassette number (Arabic numeral), and initials of the radiologic technologist who performed the examination (Fig. 3.19). The identification label should include the name and address of the facility, first and last name of examinee, and a unique identification number (e.g., medical record number, social security number, or date of birth). The technologist's initials are usually written on the identification label. The radiopaque laterality and view marker should be placed near the axilla to facilitate proper orientation of the image.

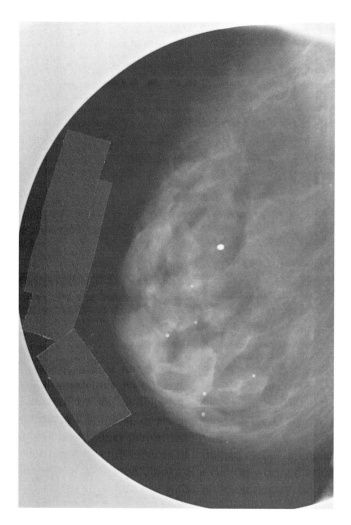

Figure 3.18. Excessive collimation of MLO view. Round collimator comes close to the surface of the breast, which makes it impossible to achieve proper viewing conditions. Axilla has been excluded from the image because of tight collimation.

Table 3.1.
Labeling Codes for Laterality and View

	Code
Right	R[a]
Left	L[a]
View	
Mediolateral oblique	MLO
Craniocaudal	CC
90° Lateral	
Mediolateral	ML
Lateromedial	LM
Magnification	M[a]
Exaggerated craniocaudal	XCCL
Cleavage	CV
Axillary tail	AT
Tangential	TAN
Roll	
Lateral	RL[b]
Medial	RM[b]
Caudocranial	FB (from below)
Lateromedial oblique	LMO
Superolateral to inferomedial oblique	SIO
Implant displaced	ID

[a]Used as a prefix before the projection; e.g., RMMLO means right magnification mediolateral oblique.

[b]Used as a suffix after the projection; e.g., LCCRL means left craniocaudal upper breast tissue rolled laterally.

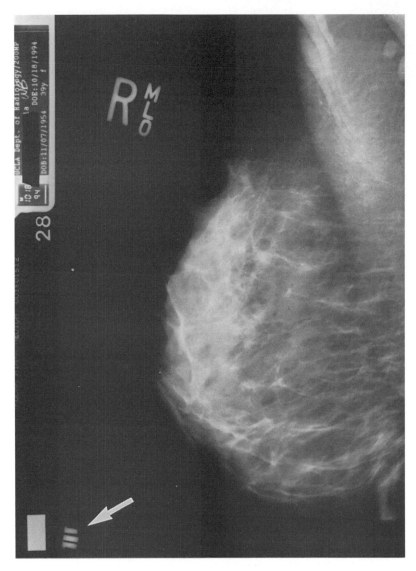

Figure 3.19. Properly labeled MLO mammogram. Patient's name on label has been masked. Radiologic technologist's initials (WB) are handwritten. The 28 identifies intensifying screen, and III (*arrow*) indicates mammography room in which the examination was performed. RMLO designates laterality and view.

Suggested Readings

American College of Radiology Committee on Quality Assurance in Mammography. Mammography quality control. Reston: American College of Radiology, 1994.

This latest version of the Mammography Quality Control manuals has a thorough section on the principles of breast positioning and film labeling. The positioning recommendations are the consensus of radiologic technologists who teach in continuing education courses for technologists.

Bassett LW, Hendrick RE, Bassford TL, et al. Quality determinants of mammography. Clinical practice guideline no. 13. Rockville MD: Agency for Health Care Policy and Research, Public Health Service, Department of Health and Human Services, Oct 1994 (AHCPR publication 95-0632).

This publication from the Agency for Health Care Policy and Research represents the combined effort of experts from different aspects of breast cancer detection, including diagnostic radiologists, medical physicists, radiologic technologists, referring health care providers, and consumer advocates. The sections on breast positioning and film labeling are pertinent to this chapter.

Bassett LW, Hirbawi IA, DeBruhl N, Hayes MK. Mammographic positioning: evaluation from the view box. Radiology 1993;188:803–806.

The article reports on the reliability of individual clinical image criteria to evaluate breast positioning; 1000 mammography examinations were performed by experienced radiologic technologists and reviewed by radiologists specializing in breast imaging. The frequency with which specific criteria were attained is reported.

Bassett LW, Jessop NW, Wilcox PA. Mammography film-labeling practices. Radiology 1993;187:773–775.

The authors report the labeling practices of mammography facilities in all regions of the United States. Recommendations for mammogram labeling are included.

PROBLEM 1

You are presented with the mammogram below from another breast imaging facility. Evaluate the film for all clinical image deficiencies. Make a list of the deficiencies, category by category, based on what you have learned in this chapter.

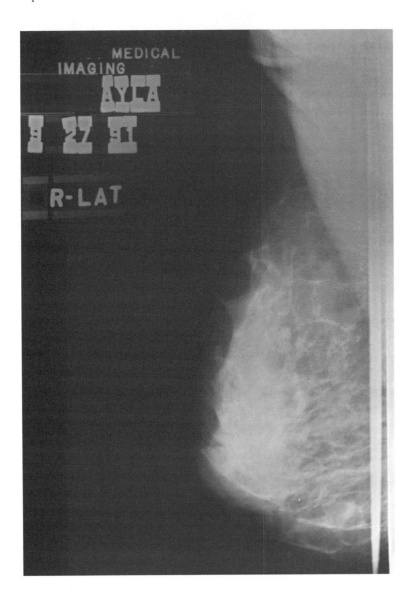

SOLUTION 1

As you go through the deficiencies found in this case, you may want to refer to Figure 3.19, which is a properly performed mammogram on the same patient performed at a different facility a few years later.

Positioning. Although a moderate amount of the pectoral muscle is included in the image, an experienced radiologic technologist could get even more muscle on the image (cf. Fig. 3.19).

Compression. The breast compression is inadequate, resulting in poor separation of the dense fibroglandular structures. There is also some blurring of the linear structures in the posterior and inferior aspects of the breast owing to motion unsharpness secondary to inadequate compression.

Exposure. The breast is underexposed based on poor visualization of details within the fibroglandular tissue and the pectoral muscle.

Contrast. There is insufficient variation in optical density when comparing the more radiolucent fatty tissue with the more radiodense fibroglandular tissue (cf. Fig. 3.19).

Sharpness. The linear structures and the edges of fibroglandular tissues are not well defined (cf. Fig. 3.19).

Artifacts. Parts of the mammography equipment are not aligned properly and are superimposed on the posterior aspect of the breast. This includes the posterior lip of the compression device and another radiopaque structure posterior to it (possibly part of the collimator or filter).

Labeling. The labeling is poor. Use of the radiopaque markers instead of a flash card identification requires a great deal more space, allows a large amount of extraneous light to pass through the film, and is distracting to the interpreting physician. The view is mislabeled (it should be "RMLO" rather than "MEDIO-LAT"). The location of the facility is not provided, increasing the likelihood that a lost film would not be returned. There is no last name and no unique identification number for the patient. The radiologic technologist is not indicated. The cassette number and room number (assuming the facility has more than one room) is not provided.

PROBLEM 2

Analyze this diagnostic mammogram of a patient with a pea-sized hard lump at 2 o'clock at the edge of the breast.

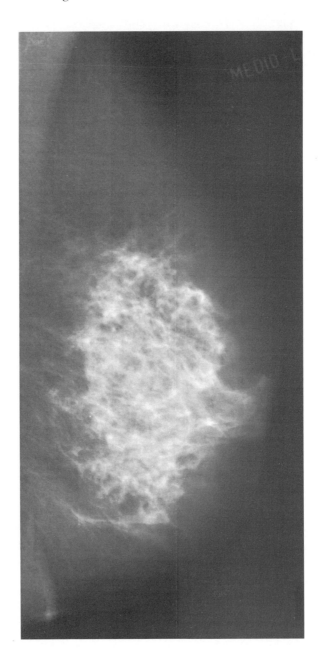

SOLUTION 2

Not enough axilla is displayed. Muscle is shown only to the top of glandular tissue. Proper positioning shows a small mass (*arrow*) with a calcification in the posterior aspect of the breast. Note that nonstandard lead marks are used.

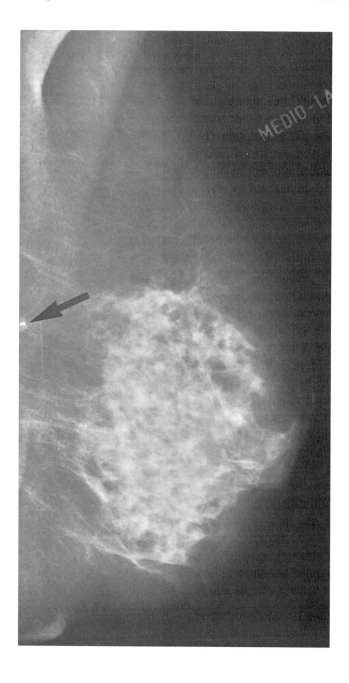

PROBLEM 3

This craniocaudal view is too light. What else is wrong with it?

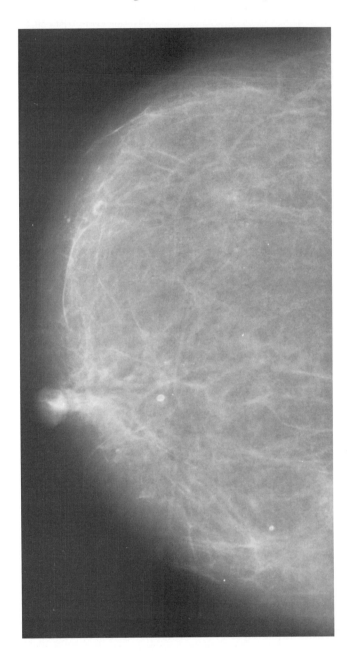

SOLUTION 3

The breast is rotated medially so that the nipple is not centered. Because medial tissue is best seen on the craniocaudal view, this mammogram has missed breast tissue particularly necessary for diagnosis.

PROBLEM 4

Muscle is well visualized to the level of the nipple; no nipple droop is present; and exposure is correct. Labels and lead marks are correct, although they have been cropped from this image. Can you explain why this film was repeated?

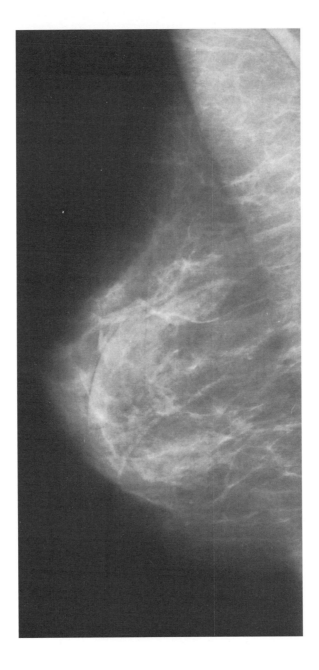

SOLUTION 4

A skin fold posterior to the nipple may conceal calcifications or breast architecture and requires correction by repeating the exposure.

QUESTIONS

1. Your facility has been asked for a second opinion for a patient whose mammograms were all underexposed. What should be done?

2. A patient has calcifications near her nipple on one view only. What should be done before this view is repeated?

3. A mass between the breasts of a patient cannot be seen on either the CC or MLO views. How can it be diagnosed?

4. If breasts are not to be collimated, how do we reduce scatter when small compression paddles are used to examine a subsection of the breast?

ANSWERS

1. Recommend that the mammograms be repeated. Because they are underexposed, contrast in glandular tissue will be poor and may mask pathology. The radiologist should not try to "read around" poor positioning and artifacts.

2. Ask the patient to wipe her breast with a towelette. Wipe down the breast support device and compression paddle. Open the cassette you plan to use and visually inspect the screen for debris. Reload the cassette, using care to touch only the film edges. If the calcifications are still present, repeat the MLO using the lateromedial oblique position.

3. See "Problem 5" in Chapter 5. A cleavage view can often resolve masses located between the breasts. A manual technique that requires lower mAs than that used for the CC view should be used because the area of interest will be thinner than the breast in the CC view.

4. We do not. We increase the dose to the breast by not collimating but improve diagnostic accuracy by using the small compression paddle so that the area of interest can be compressed more than it was when a larger compression paddle was used. We do not collimate because we want to be certain of our position in the breast and to avoid light areas around the breast when reading the film.

4

TECHNIQUES AND EQUIPMENT FOR MAMMOGRAPHICALLY GUIDED BIOPSY

A patient with a nonpalpable, mammographically detected suspicious lesion may have it localized with a hookwire by the radiologist, followed by an excision biopsy by a surgeon, or she may have a stereotactically guided core biopsy performed by the radiologist. In a facility which has the services of a trained cytopathologist, fine-needle aspiration biopsy of a clinically occult lesion that has been localized by the radiologist may be appropriate.

LOCALIZATION OF AN OCCULT LESION BEFORE SURGICAL BIOPSY

Wire placement can be performed by the biplane or stereotactic method but is much simpler by the biplane method; a stereotactic procedure is rarely used for prebiopsy localization. For the biplane method, the only special equipment required is a modified compression plate. This may be one that contains a 4 cm × 8 cm window near its posterior edge, with a lead impregnated scale on each side of the window. Alternatively, the plate may contain as many as 40 1-cm-diameter holes spaced 0.5 cm apart (Fig. 4.1). This so-called "hole plate" compresses the breast more uniformly than the compression plate with a window and does not necessitate the precise positioning required for use of the latter. However, a hole plate with 1.5-cm-diameter holes spaced widely apart is less effective than a plate with smaller, closely spaced holes because if the area of interest is located between the holes it will be more difficult to precisely localize.

Patients are usually seated during a localization procedure. If a window compression plate is used, the area of the breast to be localized is centered beneath the window, and the breast is moderately compressed in whatever projection (craniocaudal, mediolateral, or lateromedial) brings the lesion closest to the plate. After a scout mammogram has been obtained with the hole plate in place, compression of the breast is maintained while the hole most directly over the lesion is determined from the mammogram (Fig. 4.2). The skin within this hole is swabbed with betadine, and, if desired, a small amount of local anesthetic is injected intradermally. The local-

ization needle containing the hookwire is directed through the hole and inserted perpendicular to the skin all the way to its hub or until the tip is well beyond the lesion. Another mammogram is then obtained to confirm that the needle is near or superimposed on the lesion (Fig. 4.3). The hole plate is replaced with a standard compression plate, and another mammogram with the breast positioned at 90° to the first projection is obtained to show the relationship of the needle tip to the lesion. Without releasing the compression, the needle is retracted as far as necessary to place its tip at the lesion. The wire is advanced through the needle until the hook is exposed and engaged in the breast. The needle then may be removed or left in place to provide a firm, palpable land-

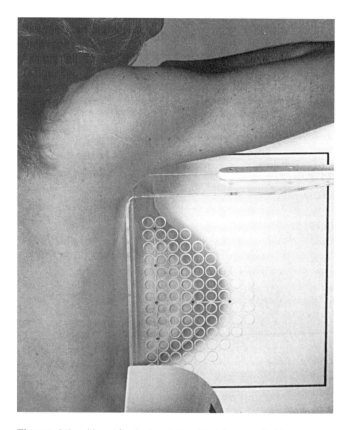

Figure 4.1. Use of a hole plate with lateromedial breast positioning.

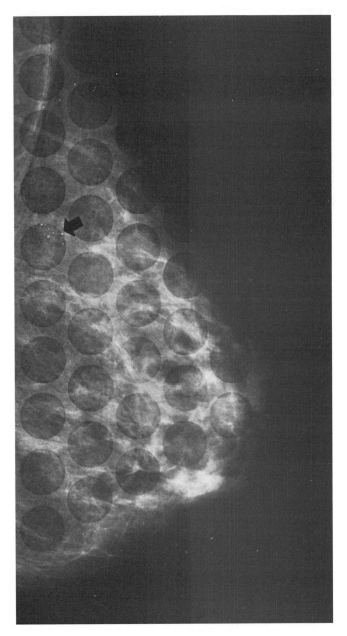

Figure 4.2. Resulting mammogram. Calcifications are seen beneath one hole in the plate (*arrow*).

mark for the surgeon. The protruding part of the wire is firmly taped to the skin. An additional pair of orthogonal radiographs is useful to confirm the close proximity of the hook of the wire to the lesion (Fig. 4.4). We consider placement to be successful when the hook is within 0.5 cm of the lesion in both craniocaudal and mediolateral (or lateromedial) projections.

Although primarily intended for fine-needle aspiration or core biopsy of clinically occult lesions, add-on stereotactic devices can also be used for prebiopsy needle localization. They are far more expensive, however, and

seem to have little if any advantage over the biplane method for prebiopsy localization.

STEREOTACTIC EQUIPMENT AND PREPARATION FOR BIOPSY

More than half of the major breast imaging centers in the United States use add-on stereotactic units or dedicated prone units (in which the patient lies prone with the breast dependent) for fine needle aspiration or core biopsies. Add-on units are a reliable option to dedicated prone units.

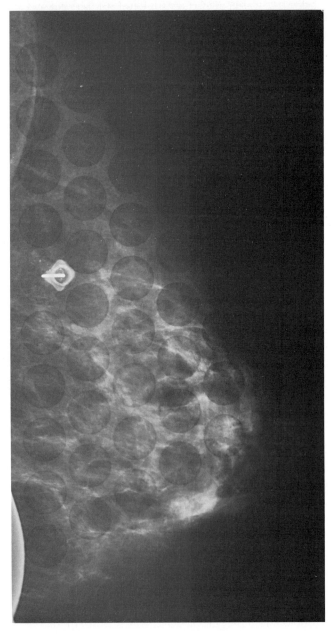

Figure 4.3. Hub of needle is seen end-on. Needle passes through the calcifications.

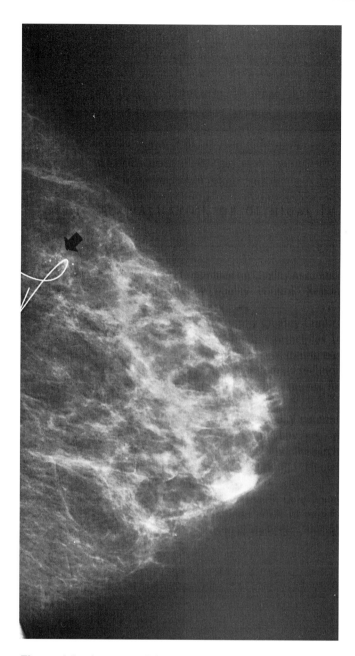

Figure 4.4. Lateromedial view with wire in place. Hook lies inferior to calcifications (*arrow*).

stereotactic viewer, which consists of a viewing screen and lesion location unit. The latter should be placed on a counter in the mammography room containing the add-on equipment. The unit that attaches to the mammography unit consists of a needle holder, a compression plate with a 5- to 6-cm square biopsy window, a film holder (with three positions for the scout, right stereo, and left stereo views), and x, y, and z knobs that move the needle into the calculated position. Modification of the mammography unit allows disengagement of the c-arm of the x-ray tube so that it can be moved 15° to 17° to the right or left of 90° without moving the film plane.

Each time the add-on stereotactic device is mounted on the mammography unit, needle calibration is performed to ensure that x, y, and z coordinates calculated for a lesion position are accurate (Fig. 4.5). First the z = 0 position is identified, as it would be during patient biopsy, by aligning the calibration needle with the corner of the compression plate. One of the following two methods of calibrating needle placement may be used: A block of plastic with holes in it is imaged stereotactically, or the needle is moved to a position inside the biopsy window and imaged stereotactically. In either case, after aligning the stereo film in the viewer, the end of a hole in the Lucite block or the tip of the needle is marked on both stereo views. Then, for calibration with the acrylic block, the needle is moved to the x, y, and z coordinates specified by the unit. If these are accurate, the needle drops into the selected hole. For the needle calibration method, the x, y, and z coordinates designated by the unit should match those of the needle position in the biopsy window.

Because clusters of calcifications as small as 3 mm in diameter may be biopsied, it is important that needle accuracy be within 2 mm. If inaccuracies during calibration are larger than 2 mm, a service engineer should be contacted, and scheduled procedures should be postponed until the unit has been repaired.

When fewer than five procedures a month are performed, an add-on unit, which is less expensive than a prone unit, can increase the accuracy of fine needle aspiration; some add-on stereotactic units can also accommodate core biopsies when the location of the lesion is such that the core needle and gun can be positioned over it.

Modifications to the mammography unit will be needed when the add-on stereotactic unit is installed. Two additional pieces of equipment are the needle holder and positioner that fit onto the mammography unit and the

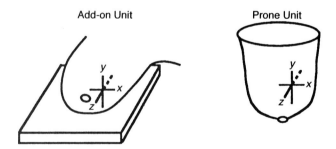

Figure 4.5. Orientation of x, y, and z coordinates to the breast.

Automatic exposure control cannot always be used for both stereo views because the needle holder covers the automatic exposure control sensor on one view. The scout view can usually be phototimed; the resulting mAs values can be used to estimate a manual technique for the stereo images.

The technologist must be certain that the needle holder and the compression paddle have been sterilized before use. As a further precaution to prevent infection, the breast support plate, *x, y,* and *z* knobs, x-ray controls, and doorknob of the procedure room should be cleaned with a disinfectant after each procedure.

STEREOTACTIC PROCEDURES

As with biplane localization, the first step in stereotactic targeting of a lesion, after mounting and calibrating the add-on component, is to position the patient so that the area of interest is centered beneath the window of the compression plate. Some add-on stereotactic units are not as accurate for laterally directed targeting as for caudally directed targeting because the former provides less breast compression and is associated with less spatial tolerance in the needle holder, allowing needle slippage. Evaluation with a gelatin training phantom will expose this source of inaccuracy. Once the location of the suspicious lesion has been verified, two stereotactic images are made on the same film. Between images, the tube is rotated 15° to 17° from the central axis, and the cassette holder is moved concurrently in the opposite direction. Automatic stops built into the device help ensure accuracy. Although the needle holder is withdrawn as much as possible to prevent it from being in the image, it may be imaged by some stereotactic systems. If the needle holder overlies the automatic exposure control sensor in the image, a manual exposure will be required.

After processing, the stereotactic radiograph is transferred to the viewer of the evaluation component of the unit. The first step in positioning the radiograph in this component is to identify landmarks common to both stereotactic views so that the coordinates, $x = 0$, $y = 0$,

$z = 0$, are identified on the film or digital image. (The *x*-axis is parallel to the chest wall side of the film, with the *y*-axis aligned in the anode-cathode direction. The *z*-axis extends between the film plane and the lesion to be sampled (Fig. 4.5). This step usually consists of lining up the radiograph along a horizontal line printed on the viewer and then aligning the vertical cursors with the crosshairs in each stereotactic image. If a digital image is available, a computer mouse is positioned on a cursor to zero-in the lesion on the localization image.

After identifying $x = 0$, $y = 0$, $z = 0$ in each image, the crosshairs are moved so that they pinpoint the lesion. The evaluation component then calculates the *x, y,* and *z* coordinates needed to localize the lesion and transmits them to the first device. The needle holder is then moved to the indicated position. The length of the needle is included in the calculations of the *z* position. The sterilized needle holder is inserted into the needle support. After sterile preparation of the skin of the breast, the needle is placed into the needle holder and introduced into the breast. To prevent movement of the needle between the needle holder and breast, the needle should fit tightly within its holder. Inaccuracies that result from inadvertent movement of the needle can be minimized by selecting the shortest needle that can reach the lesion. When the needle has been positioned, the breast, while still compressed, should again be reradiographed for pre-fire images.

DEDICATED PRONE STEREOTACTIC CORE BREAST BIOPSY

Many of these same procedures are required when using a dedicated prone stereotactic breast biopsy unit. Unlike the add-on stereotactic unit, the dedicated unit is "ready-to-go." The "under the table" configuration may seem initially to be confusing (Fig. 4.6), but after a few biopsies most users prefer not to return to an add-on unit. Patients who experience dizziness during biopsy are especially comfortable on a prone couch. The accuracy

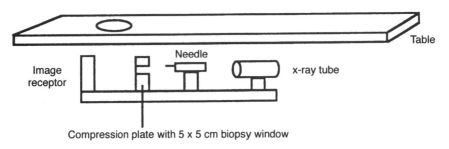

Figure 4.6. Prone stereotactic breast biopsy unit.

of needle placement must be tested each day before the first biopsy. Usually, a calibration needle is mounted in the core gun holder, and the needle method, previously described for an add-on unit, is performed. The same rigorous specifications and cleanliness requirements also apply for prone units. Most dedicated units are used only for core biopsies. The core needle (Fig. 4.7) is mounted in a spring loaded "gun." Core samples are large enough to be treated like surgical biopsy specimens. When a lesion containing calcifications is biopsied, specimen radiography should be performed on the core specimens (Fig. 4.8).

Stereotactic units can have screen/film or digital image receptors. Screen/film stereotactic units calculate the x, y, and z coordinates in the same manner that they are calculated for add-on units. Screen/film stereotactic units have either reciprocating or fixed grids. Although fixed grids are not recommended for screening or diagnostic mammography, image quality is adequate for stereotactic procedures. The fixed grid of an older stereotactic unit should be checked, at least initially, by a medical physicist who images a 2- to 4-cm thick plastic sheet to ensure that the grid is undamaged. Digital units do not require grids because contrast enhancement of the digital image restores contrast lost from scatter.

Typically, once the needle is moved to the x and y coordinates, it is advanced slowly to the aseptically prepared skin of the compressed breast. A mark is made on the skin with the tip of the needle, and this area is anesthetized. With a scalpel, the physician makes two 6-mm incisions in the form of a cross centered at the needle mark. At least five core samples are obtained, one from the center and one from each corner of the cross. For medicolegal reasons, the scout, prefire stereo, and postfire stereo views of the center core positions and the needle accuracy calibration images should be preserved on film or disk (in the case of digital image receptors) (Fig. 4.9).

DIGITAL IMAGE RECEPTORS

The primary advantage of a digital unit is that it saves time. Not only is the digital image available in 3–4 seconds, rather than 3–4 minutes for a film image, but most

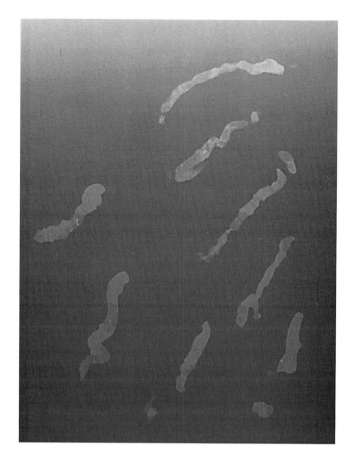

Figure 4.8. Core biopsy specimen radiograph of a cluster of calcifications.

units also transfer x and y coordinates directly from the digital workstation to the biopsy gun stage. Just as for screen/film units, the physician can still control the advancement of the needle into the breast (the z position). Some units allow the user to select either 1024×1024 resolution or 512×512 resolution. An image with higher resolution can show finer detail but requires four times more disk storage than the lower resolution image. When a cluster of microcalcifications is being biopsied, the higher resolution image may be needed for the scout view to identify the calcifications. Automatic exposure control is available with screen/film systems but not with all digital systems. Digital units allow greater exposure latitude; because contrast can be manipulated digitally by the technologist, very low exposures may still provide a reasonable image of a mass. For microcalcifications, however, a low exposure may produce such a noisy image that calcifications are obscured. If a scout view of a focus of known calcifications does not match prebiopsy screen/film views, the technique should be adjusted. The rule of doubling the mAs for each centimeter of compressed breast tissue is useful here. If the

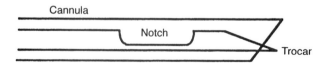

Figure 4.7. Core needle (14 gauge).

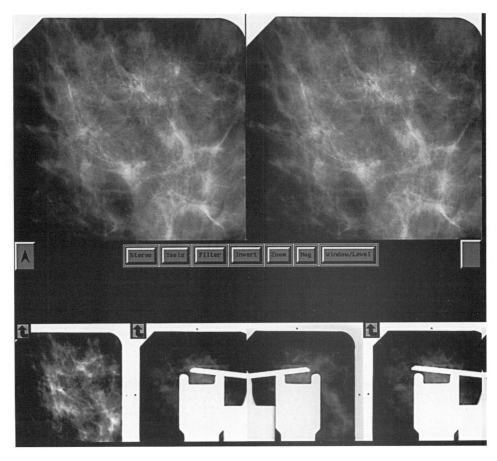

Figure 4.9. Digital stereotactic breast biopsy images on a dedicated prone unit. *Bottom left*, scout view; *top*, stereo views; *bottom middle*, prefire; *bottom right*, postfire.

American College of Radiology (ACR) mammography accreditation phantom, at 4.5 cm thickness, is successfully imaged using 512 × 512 resolution at 28 kVp, 48 mAs, then a 5.5-cm-thick compressed breast will require 96 mAs. Furthermore, if 1024 × 1024 resolution is used to localize calcifications in the 5.5-cm-thick breast, at least 192 mAs will be needed. An applications specialist can provide specific recommendations for the particular system.

AMERICAN COLLEGE OF RADIOLOGY ACCREDITATION

The procedure for accreditation of stereotactic units is similar to that for mammography accreditation. However, because digital units have a limited field of view (usually 5 × 5 cm), obtaining images of the ACR mammography phantom may present a special problem because four images are needed. Smaller calibration phantoms are available for stereotactic units and are recommended. In addition, a gelatin phantom with embedded targets can

be made or purchased to test the accuracy of the equipment and of the physicians performing the procedure before it is attempted on patients.

SPECIMEN RADIOGRAPHY

All surgical biopsies of the breast and core biopsies of lesions containing microcalcifications should be followed by specimen radiography. The purpose of specimen radiography is to verify that the mammographic abnormality has been included in the excised tissue and to pinpoint the most suspicious focus for the pathologist (Fig. 4.8). Although specimen radiographs can be performed with conventional mammography equipment, to avoid interruption of the flow of patients it is convenient to use a small, self-contained dedicated x-ray unit for the task. The specimen(s) and accompanying radiograph are taken to the pathologist for correlative histologic examination. Masses and architectural distortion on occasion may be difficult to appreciate in specimen radiographs despite the use of various projections, compression of the specimen, and magnification films. In these cases, mammograms should be repeated within approximately 2 months to ensure that the lesion was removed.

If conventional mammographic equipment is used, it is preferable to perform specimen radiography with the lowest kVp setting available, manual technique, and magnification with the small focal spot. No grid should be used because the small amount of tissue in the specimen will generate only minimal scatter, and the short exposure may result in grid lines that degrade the image. If the mammography unit cannot make a short enough exposure to radiograph the specimen, place a 0.5- to 1.0-cm-thick block of plastic on the specimen during the exposure. The combination usually can be imaged satisfactorily between 4 and 8 mAs, depending on the SID and mR/mAs. One type of dedicated stereotactic breast biopsy unit has a specimen holder that allows the unit to image core samples.

The dedicated specimen x-ray units of different manufacturers are similar. The specimen may be placed on a piece of clear film that is then placed directly on the film-screen cassette. A 3- to 10-second exposure at 18 kVp is adequate for most small specimens. Large specimens may require compression with a thin sheet of plastic weighted on its four corners by pieces of lead.

Suggested Readings

Bassett LW, Jackson VP, Jahan R, Fu YS, Gold RH. Diagnosis of diseases of the breast. Philadelphia: Saunders, 1996: Chapters 16, 17, 19, 20.

All interventional procedures requiring breast imaging are covered and are addressed primarily to physicians.

Hendrick RE, Parker SH. Principles of stereotactic mammography and quality assurance. In Parker SH, Joby WE, eds. Percutaneous breast biopsy. New York: Raven, 1993.

This chapter describes the step-by-step procedure required for stereotactic localization, provides the formulas necessary to calculate the coordinates of the lesion, and lists possible sources of error.

Kimme-Smith C, Solberg T. Acceptance testing prone stereotactic breast biopsy units. Med Physics 1994;21:1197–1201.

Some difficulties medical physicists may encounter when acceptance-testing dedicated stereotactic units are described. It is intended primarily for medical physicists familiar with Mammography Quality Standards Act mammography surveys.

PROBLEM 1

A mass viewed on both craniocaudal (**A**) and mediolateral (**B**) projections was successfully localized (*arrows*) in the mediolateral projection. After breast compression was released, the craniocaudal projection no longer showed the mass. What is the explanation?

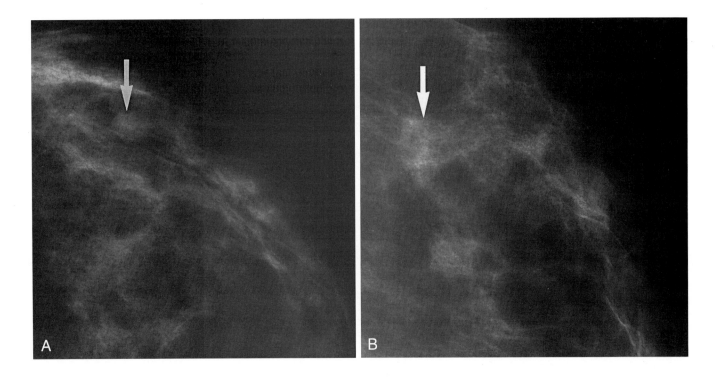

SOLUTION 1

The mass was a cyst. When it was pierced by the localization needle, the fluid in the cyst drained out, decompressing it, and resulting in its disappearance.

PROBLEM 2

After prebiopsy localization, a specimen radiograph failed to show the focus of calcifications that was the object of investigation. The surgeon doubts that she missed the lesion which the radiologist believed was accurately localized. Is there any other possible explanation?

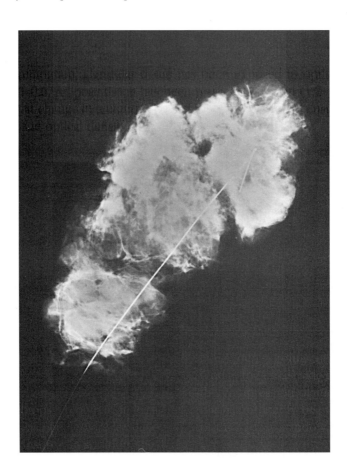

SOLUTION 2

The specimen radiograph was underexposed. When the technique was corrected, the calcifications were seen in the specimen.

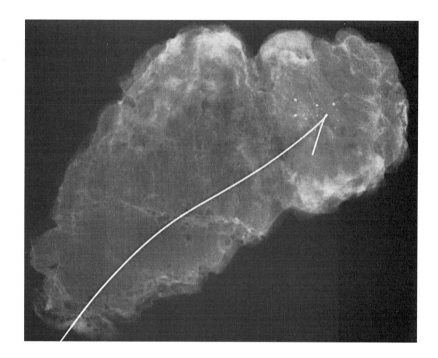

PROBLEM 3

The ACR mammography accreditation phantom was imaged with the digital image receptor using the same technique that was used for screen/film: 28 kVp, 32 mAs. The drawing shows the positioning of the phantom in the 5 × 5 cm biopsy window. Does the image meet expectations for image quality?

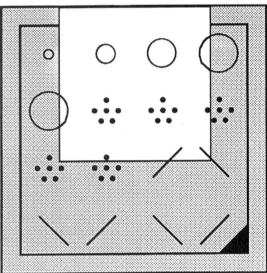

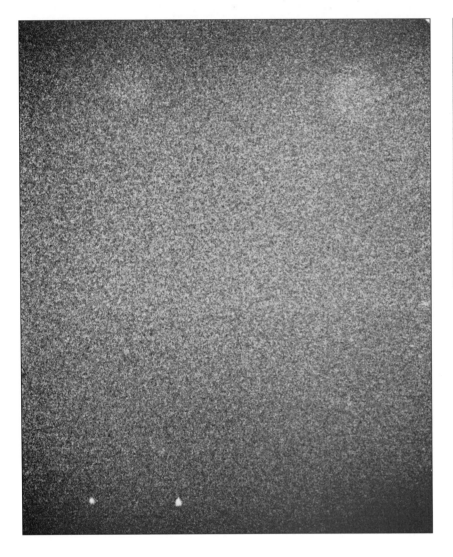

SOLUTION 3

No. On digital systems the fourth set of specks should have been visible, as they are in the image below, when 96 mAs was the setting. Note that mean glandular dose is still low for this exposure: 165 mrad.

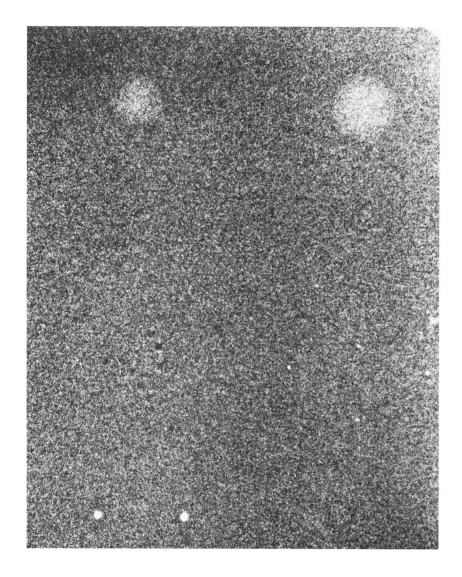

PROBLEM 4

The physicist measured the focal spot resolution of the digital receptor for the prone stereotactic unit with a line pair phantom and reported that a resolution of only 5 line pairs/mm (see line pair image below), far below the minimum required by the ACR. Should the unit be rejected?

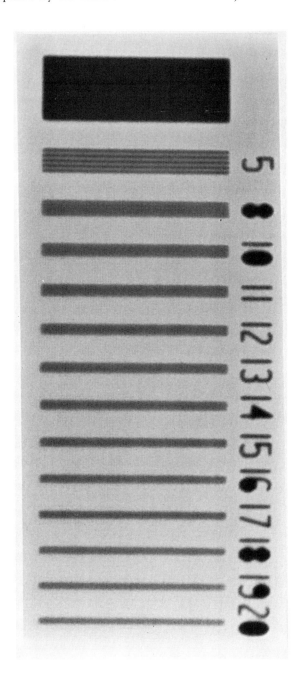

SOLUTION 4

No. The physicist measured the line pair phantom using the digital system, which has a limiting resolution of about 7.5 line pairs/mm in the 1024 × 1024 mode. The physicist measured the digital receptor rather than the focal spot. When a screen/film was placed behind the phantom (see below), the resolution was 13 line pairs/mm. For systems with fixed grids, the screen/film cassette should be placed in front of the fixed grid because grid lines will interfere with interpretation of the phantom image.

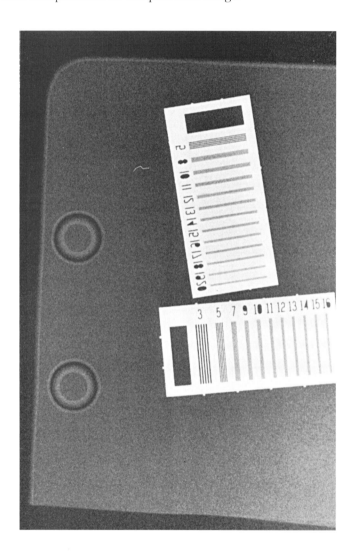

QUESTIONS

1. Because a patient with a cluster of suspicious calcifications (BI RADS category 4) is concerned about the radiation dose, she refuses a stereotactically guided core biopsy using a digital receptor. Instead, she elects localization with a hole plate followed by open biopsy. Because localization also requires x-ray exposure, has she saved herself any radiation exposure by this decision?

2. You notice that the masses imaged on your stereotactic unit shift to the right or left but never up or down in the stereo images. Is your unit operating correctly?

3. During needle accuracy calibration, the needle position is never calculated to be as deep as it actually is. Should the service engineer be called if the inaccuracy is 3 mm?

4. After a service engineer performed routine preventive maintenance on the digital stereo unit, none of the images could be recalled. What caused this problem?

5. During fine needle aspiration using the stereotactic add-on unit, the needle wobbles in the needle support device, and the x, y deflection at the lesion is much more than 2 mm. What is wrong?

ANSWERS

1. Yes. The stereotactic core biopsy requires at least seven x-ray exposures, whereas needle/wire localization requires at least four exposures. In addition, digital imaging of calcifications requires about two to three times the radiation required for screen/film images. This may change when more sensitive digital receptors have been developed.

2. Yes. Only the x direction location changes because the stereo shift is only in the x direction. If the lesion was lower in one stereo view, the patient must have shifted her position between the two views.

3. No. When zeroing the needle, the point should extend to the breast side of the biopsy window. Because the compression plate is about 3 mm thick, the needle has probably been zeroed to the x-ray tube side of the biopsy window.

4. The service engineer has transferred the hard disk images to the optical disk. If you wish to recall them, they have to be transferred back to the hard disk of the workstation.

5. Either the needle holder does not fit the needle gauge, or the second needle support is not sufficiently separated from the first needle support to stabilize the needle. This is a common problem of some add-on units.

5

AUTOMATIC EXPOSURE CONTROL

Automatic exposure control (AEC) for mammography is particularly necessary because of the high contrast film needed for good mammography images. Whenever contrast is high, image latitude is reduced. It is this reduction in latitude that makes accurate phototiming so critical in mammography. Small changes in radiation exposure can make the difference between a diagnostic mammogram and one that will result in a misdiagnosis. Exposure sensors for mammography have not always worked as reliably as they do in today's state-of-the-art machines. Current mammography equipment can now be expected to respond dependably, with less than 0.24 optical density variation between films over a range of mammographic energies and breast thicknesses.

A mammography AEC consists of a solid state detector placed under the screen/film cassette, an amplifier, a voltage comparator, and an exposure terminator (Fig. 5.1).

The sensor is typically a single large (10 cm²) detector or an array of three or more small (1 cm²) detectors. The sensor can be moved back and forth, enabling it to be positioned under the glandular region of the breast. If an array of detectors is used, a computer algorithm may determine the glandular region. When installed, the AEC is adjusted by the manufacturer's service engineer. The screen/film combination, film processor parameters, and desired film density all affect AEC calibration. It is the physicist's responsibility to verify during acceptance testing that the AEC density setting is correct.

ACCEPTANCE TESTING

A stack of different thicknesses of tissue-equivalent material is required to test the AEC device. Composites such as BR12 or similar epoxies that represent a 50% glandular/50% adipose breast mixture are preferred. If these are

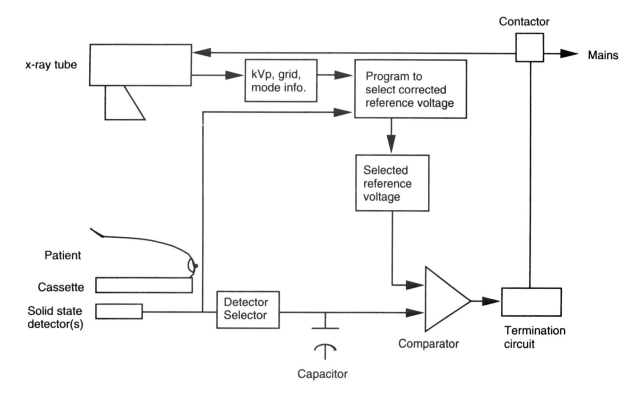

Figure 5.1. Typical AEC circuit.

unobtainable, an acrylic substitute such as Lucite can be used, but it may not satisfactorily represent fatty breasts compressed to less than a 4-cm thickness for any exposure made with < 28 kVp. If BR12 was not used to calibrate the AEC, the technologist may have to reduce the AEC control by one density setting for small breasts to avoid producing an overexposed radiograph.

During acceptance testing, density tracking for test object thicknesses between 2 and 6 cm should be checked at 2-cm increments for the commonly used kVps. For some older, underpowered units, grid exposures for breasts thicker than 6 cm may not be possible without the unit "timing out." In those situations, kVp will have to be increased. A well-designed mammography unit provides the automatic selection of different AEC settings according to whether nongrid, grid, or magnification techniques are being used. In several older units, AEC settings for these different techniques must be selected manually. The AEC density tracking of various breast (phantom) thicknesses should be tested for the different techniques over the range of kVps used. Because a 6-cm thick breast would be coned and compressed on magnified views to a smaller thickness (e.g., 4 cm), magnification AEC performance can be tested over a 2- to 4-cm range. For magnification, a grid should not be used, and x-ray tube potential is generally 2 kVp higher than that used for grid mammography. Because some manufacturers use the position of the compression device to help predict the correct AEC exposure, it is important during acceptance testing that the compression paddle lay directly on top of the breast phantom.

Although AEC exposure reproducibility is generally not a problem with state-of-the-art units, it nevertheless should be checked when the unit is new to establish the range of variation. In addition to the above, AEC acceptance testing also should include a determination of the percentage exposure (mAs) change associated with the AEC ± density settings. The density setting will be used rarely in a properly functioning facility. When the AEC meets the Mammography Quality Standards Act standards of density tracking across different breast thicknesses and when processing and film speed are controlled by daily sensitometry, changes in the density setting are not necessary. However, occasional patients have very glandular breasts that may attenuate the x-ray beam more than expected, or new film types may be tested at the facility. For these reasons, density variations should be available. Because these problems can usually be compensated for by changing the density setting on the AEC control by one or two steps, it is important to determine

during acceptance testing if the AEC density control performs in an acceptable manner. It is desirable to have a wide range of AEC density steps available (e.g., −5, −4, −3, −2, −1, 0, +1, +2, +3, +4, +5). Each AEC step should alter the AEC exposure by 10–15%.

AEC EXPOSURE TERMINATION

Because many mammography equipment manufacturers have recently modified their AEC devices to improve the consistency of film exposures, they may use the improved AEC design as a feature to publicize their equipment. A review of some of the problems associated with breast phototiming may help the user understand why some AEC devices function better than others. The sensitivity of the sensors used to generate a current during an exposure varies directly with kVp. Because the dialed kVp can be included in the computer program that terminates the exposure, this change in sensitivity of the sensor cell can be compensated for by a built-in table that lists termination values for each kVp in the exposure termination computer program. Because the low kVp settings used in mammography result in the breast absorbing more low than high energy photons, the photons that reach the AEC sensor cells will consist of fewer low than high energy photons. The proportion of low and high energy photons that reaches the AEC sensors depends on the thickness and glandular content of the breast. Sampling the photons for their energy mixture after they have passed through the breast, therefore, can help stabilize AEC exposures.

Another dilemma of mammography exposure control is that the small focal spots and low kVp techniques require long exposures, sometimes more than 2 seconds. Films exposed to light photons from screens react nonlinearly to long exposures; i.e., the same number of light photons delivered during a short interval (between 0.05 and 0.5 seconds) and during a long interval (between 1.0 and 3.0 seconds) will produce different film darkening. This effect, called "film reciprocity law failure," can cause premature exposure termination for thick or very dense breasts. Manufacturers have attempted to compensate for this error by various methods. One solution is for the unit to sense the thickness of the compressed breast by the position of the compression paddle and to modify the exposure termination program accordingly. Another technique presamples the breast with a short test exposure just before the imaging exposure. The number of photons that reaches the sensor during the test exposure determines the cut-off voltage for the imaging exposure. Yet a third method adds extra time to the longer exposures, whereas short exposures terminate without any adjustment.

Another problem is caused by heterogeneous breast parenchyma. Because the sensor cell covers a finite area that may lie beneath fatty or glandular tissue, overexposure or underexposure may result in areas of the breast not directly over the sensor. If the patient's previous radiographs are available, and if they show that the parenchyma overlying the usual sensor position is fatty whereas the more anterior parenchyma is glandular, then the sensor position should be adjusted by the technologist so that it lies beneath the glandular tissue. Some machines contain multiple sensors or an array of sensors that terminate the exposure when the sensor with the least voltage has accumulated a threshold voltage.

The introduction of beam hardening filters such as Rh, as well as Rh or W anode materials, has complicated AEC termination algorithms. Many manufacturers now provide phototimers that select anode, filter, and kVp based on breast thickness or presampled exposure of the compressed breast. These algorithms may be based on laboratory measurements of breast phantoms that do not simulate clinical experience. Recent statistical surveys of glandular content in breasts have shown that as compressed breast thickness increases, the percentage of glandular tissue decreases (see Grise and Palchevsky under "Suggested Readings"). However, most AEC tests are performed with phantoms that are assumed to contain a combination of 50% glandular tissue-equivalent material and 50% adipose tissue-equivalent material. Thus the kVp and anode material recommended by the AEC may be inappropriate. In general, these programs do not recommend using Rh or W anodes unless breast thickness is 6 cm or greater, and then the kVp recommended is higher than is consistent with good contrast. For these reasons, selection of anode and filter material, as well as of kVp, may more appropriately be made by an experienced technologist who has access to the patient's previous films.

AUTOMATIC EXPOSURE CONTROL PROBLEMS

Many problems can arise during routine use of AEC devices. Some of these problems can be corrected by the technologist, whereas others will require the assistance of a service engineer, and some are inherent in the equipment.

The most common reason for underexposure of a film is that the AEC sensor is incorrectly placed. When a large-breasted patient is followed by a small-breasted patient, the technologist may forget to readjust the sensor to the more posterior position. Even more frequently, the sensor is inadvertently left near the chest wall and not repositioned under the glandular tissue of a large-breasted woman. This error produces underexposure of the glandular portion of the breast. Even though radiologists' preferences vary, most correctly exposed mammograms range from optical densities of 0.6–1.2 for glandular tissue and 1.2–2.2 for fatty tissue. When glandular tissue is exposed to < 0.6 optical density, contrast may be too low to recognize pathology. For this reason, glandular parenchyma should always be exposed to a medium gray value.

Occasionally, oblique views include so much muscle over the AEC that the breast tissue is overexposed. This is because the AEC was calibrated by using breast-equivalent material and the pectoral muscle tissue, which attenuates the x-rays even more, changes the exposure termination factors. In that situation, the sensor should be moved anteriorly so that it is positioned under the breast tissue. Another problem common to many AEC devices is underexposure of very small, dense breasts. Even when the breast seems to cover the sensor (as indicated by the compression paddle locator), scatter from the film holder near the skin can terminate the exposure prematurely. For these patients, manual techniques are needed.

The above problems can be solved by the technologist. Other problems require the aid of a service engineer. If the AEC underexposes or overexposes every mammogram, and film/processor quality control assessments show that these factors are unchanged compared with previous values, then changing the AEC density setting should be considered a temporary solution. If acceptance testing verified optical density tracking with changes in kVp, then changing the kVp should not affect film darkening when the projection is repeated at different kVps. The service engineer should determine if the dialed kVp is consistent with that actually delivered. Repeated AEC exposures of the same breast in the same projection may be necessary during prebiopsy localization and should not vary visibly in optical density. Should the optical density vary, multiple images of a mammography phantom will reveal whether the AEC is functioning consistently. The service engineer should be consulted if repeated phantom images vary more than 0.1 optical density when measured at the same position on the radiograph.

Intermittent AEC malfunction is as difficult to identify as it is to rectify. Because of the expense of service by the manufacturer, every effort should be made to discover and correct AEC problems while the mammography unit is still under warranty.

Suggested Readings

Grise RA, Palchevsky A. Composition of mammographic phantom materials. Radiology 1996;198:347–350.

This research paper indicates the problems that physicists encounter when simulating clinical breast composition to test AEC devices.

Krestel E. Imaging systems for medical diagnostics. Berlin: Siemens, 1990:302–305.

This short section of a complex text gives circuit diagrams and equations that are useful for exposure control.

Thompson TT. A practical approach to modern imaging equipment, 2nd ed. Boston: Little Brown, 1985:130–137.

This gives a detailed, readable presentation of AEC methods for all types of radiographic procedures. It is the only reference that discusses solid state detectors in the context of radiographic density control.

PROBLEM 1

For this mammogram, glandular tissue has been exposed to optical density values of 0.3–0.6. Adipose tissue has been properly exposed (1.2–1.6 optical density). What change in technique would you recommend to ensure correct glandular tissue optical density?

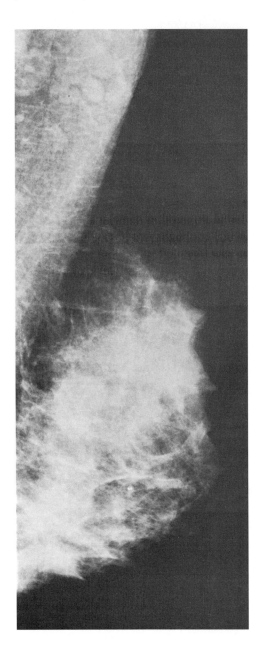

SOLUTION 1

Place the AEC sensor under the glandular tissue in the breast. The image below illustrates the correct exposure.

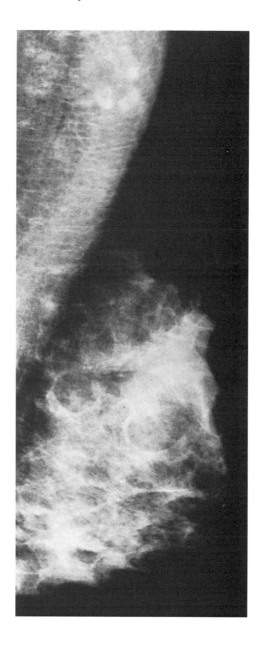

PROBLEM 2

This breast image is underexposed, yet the AEC sensor was completely covered by breast tissue. What went wrong?

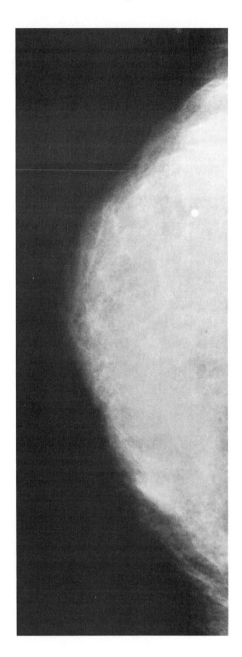

SOLUTION 2

The AEC sensor of this unit extends 4 cm from the chest wall, but the breast extends only to 4.5 cm from the chest wall. The small amount of tissue at the nipple is not enough attenuation to prevent premature AEC termination. When a manual exposure is performed, the breast is correctly exposed. If a breast imaging center has only one mammography unit, the AEC of that unit must be able to permit small breasts to be imaged correctly.

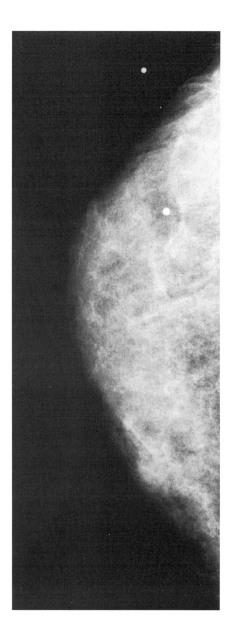

PROBLEM 3

This encapsulated silicon implant cannot be imaged with the Eklund implant displacement technique. Where should the AEC be placed to prevent over-exposure?

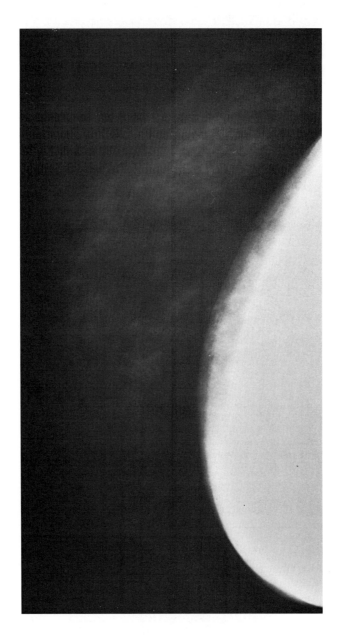

SOLUTION 3

Manual exposure is necessary. When the silicon implant is imaged, do not try to predict its position with respect to the AEC sensor.

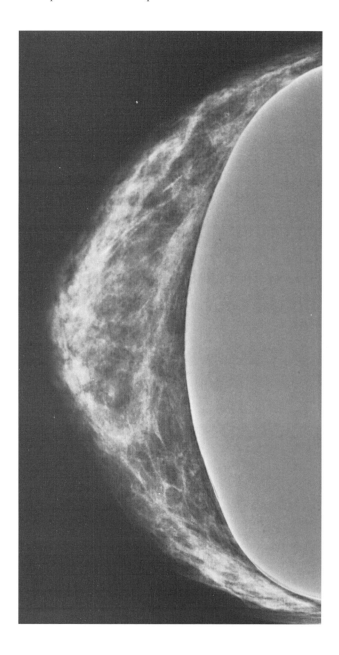

PROBLEM 4

Although the magnified views of this breast were consistently overexposed, the physicist found that the AEC worked correctly for the magnified views. What could have happened?

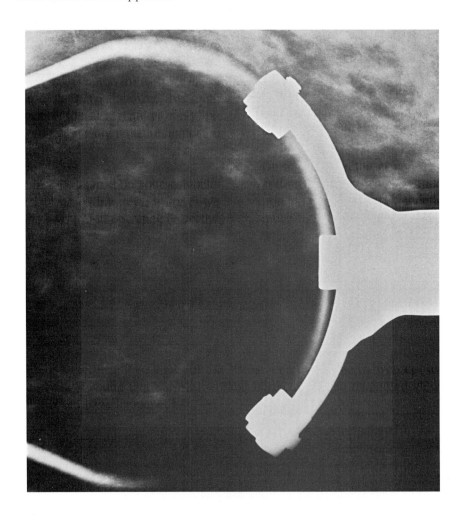

SOLUTION 4

The AEC sensor is not under the tissue but is being partially blocked by the compression paddle support. The sensor should be moved closer to the chest wall.

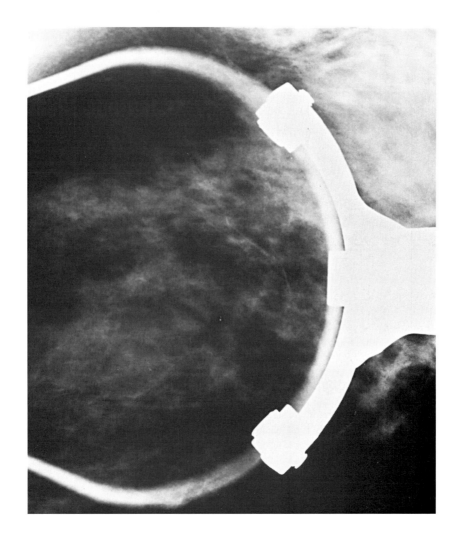

PROBLEM 5

What is the image below? What was the purpose of the image? Was it successful?

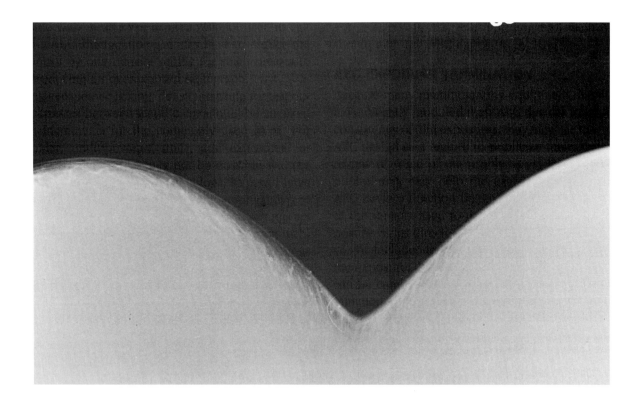

SOLUTION 5

This is a cleavage view performed to image a mass located near the chest wall between the breasts. Because the AEC sensor was not covered by breast tissue, the image was underexposed. This is another example of a view that requires a manual exposure.

QUESTIONS

1. If the AEC terminates after it receives a certain exposure, why is the glandular tissue overlying the sensor not exposed to the same optical density to which the adipose tissue overlying the sensor is exposed?

2. A coned down, collimated view of a breast abnormality requires more exposure, using the AEC, than a noncollimated AEC view of the same abnormality. The resulting images have the same optical density. What accounts for this difference in AEC performance?

3. Why do craniocaudal views require less exposure than mediolateral oblique views of the same breast when the optical density of the two views is equivalent?

4. Why are magnified views obtained using the AEC so often lighter in optical density than nonmagnified views?

5. To image a predominantly fatty breast that contains an area of postradiotherapy fibrosis posterior to the nipple, should the AEC sensor be placed under the area of fibrosis?

6. A large dense breast was imaged at 26 kVp with a +2 density setting on a Mo anode unit. What density setting should be used when imaging the same breast at the same kVp with a Rh anode unit?

ANSWERS

1. The energy spectra exiting from the glandular tissue will be harder (there will be fewer low energy photons) than the energy spectra exiting from the adipose tissue. Because solid state detectors are more sensitive to higher energy photons, they will terminate sooner when the AEC sensor is under glandular tissue. Thus the film will be lighter in optical density than it would have been had the AEC sensor been located under adipose tissue.

2. Because the collimated view has less scatter from surrounding tissue than the uncollimated view, there is less film darkening. Therefore, the exposure must be greater to achieve the same optical density as achieved by the uncollimated view.

3. The mediolateral oblique projection images the pectoralis muscle, which prevents compression of the breast to the same thickness that can be achieved in the craniocaudal projection. A thicker compressed breast requires more exposure.

4. Although the AEC should compensate for this difference, not all of them do. The difference in optical density is due to the difference in energy spectrum between magnified and nonmagnified views. This energy difference can be due to difference in technique (magnified views are usually obtained at higher kVp than nonmagnified views) or attenuation of low energy photons in the air gap. Because the AEC sensor is more sensitive to high energy photons, the exposure may terminate prematurely.

5. It may be necessary to obtain two views of the breast in the same projection. The fibrosis will be more attenuating and may be underexposed if the AEC sensor is not placed under it. Optimally exposed views of this area will assist in the identification of recurrent cancer. However, the surrounding adipose tissue will be overexposed. Therefore additional views of the breast with the AEC sensor placed subjacent to the adipose tissue may be needed to obtain diagnostic optical densities of the untreated part of the breast.

6. If the AEC program has been calibrated, the same density setting should be used for the Rh anode. In practice, however, a +1 density setting is usually sufficient because of the greater penetration of the Rh energy spectrum.

6

RESOLUTION

Before the 1970s, intensifying screens that provided a combination of high sensitivity and fine detail for mammography were unavailable. Instead, high-resolution industrial film was used, resulting in large radiation dosages. In the same era, resolution was degraded by large focal spots, short source-to-image distances (SID), and absent or inadequate compression. The high resolution of industrial film was wasted because of the poor geometric unsharpness inherent in the mammography equipment at that time. The matching of excellent image receptor resolution and improved geometric resolution occurred about 20 years ago, when engineering science was applied to mammography as a total system rather than by piecemeal evaluation of its component parts. High resolution capability of screen/film combinations was coupled with smaller focal spot size and reduced object magnification (determined by the distances between the focal spot and breast and between the breast and image receptor).

Current mammography screen/film combinations must be able to image a high contrast test object (see under "Problem 5" in Chapter 4) so that 13 line pairs/mm can be seen with a magnifying lens. Lower contrast test objects, such as simulated calcifications embedded in a block of acrylic, cannot be seen as accurately. In fact, calcifications smaller than 0.2 mm (2.5 line pairs/mm) can rarely be imaged by screen/film mammographic systems if the usual scatter and magnification are present.

FOCAL SPOT SIZE AND SID

Focal spot size and the amount of magnification of the object determine geometric resolution. Because magnification depends on the ratio of the distances between the focal spot and the object of interest compared with the distance between the object of interest and the image receptor, resolution is affected by SID, compression, and location in the breast of the area of interest. The size of the focal spot will affect the amount of blur at the edge of the object of interest. If the blur is bigger than half the object diameter, contrast will be less than it would have been for a larger object, a smaller focal spot, or less magnification, and our chances of detecting it are reduced.

Older equipment may have SIDs shorter than 60 cm, but all mammography equipment manufactured since 1992 has SIDs of 60, 65, or 76 cm. Focal spot size for contact mammograms must be small enough to ensure that 13 line pairs/mm can be seen on an image of a high contrast test object placed 4.5 cm above the image receptor. This can usually be accomplished by a focal spot whose actual (not nominal) size is < 0.45 mm wide. This limitation implies a nominal focal spot size of 0.3 mm. Similarly, microfocal magnification mammography with a 1.5× stand should not be attempted for short SID systems unless the actual size of the width of the small focal spot is ≤0.2 mm.

FOCAL SPOT MEASUREMENTS

Some confusion may exist about the techniques of measuring a focal spot in order to obtain its "actual" width. The width of a focal spot refers to its size when measured perpendicular to the anode-cathode direction. Because all mammography units mount the cathode nearest the patient and the anode nearest the body of the x-ray unit (Fig. 6.1), the width of the focal spot is measured from the patient's left to right. Focal spot width does not vary when measured near the chest wall or near the nipple at the center line but can vary slightly if measured to the right or left of the center line. A 0.01-mm slit is needed to measure the size of focal spots. It is difficult to position the slit in the "central ray" so that the edges of the slit do not block x-rays and give spurious measurements of the focal spot size. Pinhole images (made with a 0.03-mm aperture) allow the physicist to assess the shape of the focal spot. One manufacturer has replaced filament cathodes with planar electron emitters that should be checked with a pinhole image during acceptance testing (Fig. 6.2). In fact, it is helpful to obtain a pinhole image if the focal spot is either innovative or if it is biased by externally applied voltage. Because ex-

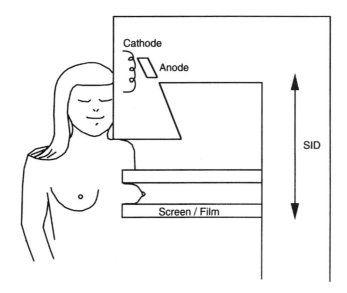

Figure 6.1. Relationship of patient to x-ray tube orientation. Placing the cathode near the chest wall increases penetration there because of the heel effect.

ternally applied biasing voltage may vary with the age of the unit or with other factors, tubes whose biasing voltage can be adjusted are more likely to have distorted focal spots.

Finally, the length of the focal spot may vary by as much as two times between the chest wall and nipple for some anode and tube-tilt angles (Fig. 6.3). Although at the nipple, focal spot length is generally about the same as its width, near the chest wall the focal spot is elongated. The resultant distortion is minimal for contact breast imaging; however, to avoid distortion on magnification images, microfocal spots tend to be square rather than rectangular.

MOTION

Once the correct focal spot size has been selected and tested for the SID of a particular mammography unit, the focal spot is unlikely to undergo significant change during the life of the x-ray tube. Resolution is more apt to be degraded because of patient motion caused by inadequate compression or excessively long exposures. When compression is firm, motion is unlikely to occur if the patient is cooperative and the time of exposure is under 1 second. Long exposures are usually attributable to underpowered systems or to microfocal magnification views of compressed breasts thicker than 5 cm. An underpowered mammography unit cannot properly expose a

compressed 5-cm thick breast in < 1 second. Even when the patient holds her breath, heartbeat and involuntary motion may affect resolution. The microfocal spot used for magnification mammography may reduce mA output by one-fourth that of the large focal spot. An exposure four times that used for a contact view, therefore, will be needed for a microfocal magnification image if all other factors remain the same. To reduce the exposure time (and therefore the dose received by the patient) for microfocal spot magnification images, three techniques can be used:

1. The kVp can be increased by 2 kVp over that of a contact view. This increases mR/mAs and also can increase the number of higher energy photons that reach the image receptor through the air gap used for magnification. Contrast will not be affected as adversely as it would be for a contact image obtained at 2 kVp higher because the air gap of the magnified view will attenuate low keV scattered photons. If a Rh filter or a Rh anode is available, their use will reduce exposure time by 20–40% compared with a Mo filter and Mo anode.
2. The breast can be spot-compressed with a compression plate about 4 cm in diameter. The compression device is positioned over the area of interest. Because compression is not applied to the whole breast, a much thinner segment of compressed breast results. For each centimeter of added compression compared with whole breast compression, exposure time can be reduced by 50%.

Figure 6.2. Instead of a coil for the cathode, this manufacturer has a plane emitter, which has an intensity distribution very different from a conventional cathode. With permission of Radiological Clinics of North America (1992) 30:56.

3. A grid should not be used. By not using a grid, exposure time can be reduced by 50%. For long SID units, scatter is reduced by the air gap between the breast and image receptor almost as effectively as with a grid, although attenuation in air of the primary photons also increases the exposure needed so that dose is only slightly less than that required by a contact view with a grid.

GRIDS AND RESOLUTION

Fixed grids (80 lines/cm) interfere with the recognition and analysis of fine microcalcifications and should not be used for mammography. Reciprocating grids (3.5:1 to 5:1, 27–46 lines/cm) can interfere with the detection of calcifications if they are not operating correctly. Any hint of grid lines in a mammogram indicates grid malfunc-

tion. The grid lines of a reciprocating grid are more likely to be seen when a small-breasted woman is imaged in a lateral or oblique projection.

CONTRAST AND RESOLUTION

Earlier, we described the differences between the resolution achievable with high contrast and low contrast test objects. Many problems diagnosed as resolution failures are really contrast failures. Once the focal spot has been measured and found to be within specification, compression, motion, and grid movement should be checked. If these are not contributing to loss of resolution, insufficient contrast should be suspected. As a practical point, poor contrast is more likely to cause loss of resolution than any geometric factor discussed in this chapter.

Information obtained from a modulation transfer function curve (Fig. 6.4) clarifies the trade-off between resolution and contrast. This curve maps the frequency, or line pairs/mm, that can be perceived on the abscissa (x) axis and the contrast (or power) on the ordinate (y) axis. At 100% contrast, where $y = 0$, an "infinite" number of line pairs/mm is seen. As contrast decreases (moving up the ordinate scale), a decreasing number of line pairs/mm is seen. The modulation transfer function curve changes when magnification or motion is introduced because these two conditions reduce the number of identifiable line pairs/mm.

Although contrast is usually associated with film darkening, contrast also depends on the ratio of optical densities between the object we wish to see and the background that surrounds the object (see Chapter 7). This

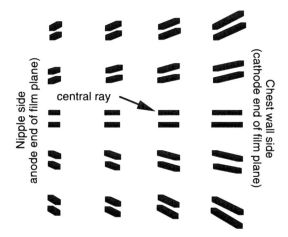

Figure 6.3. Variation of focal spot size with position in the anode-cathode direction. Central ray is measured at the chest wall in the center position.

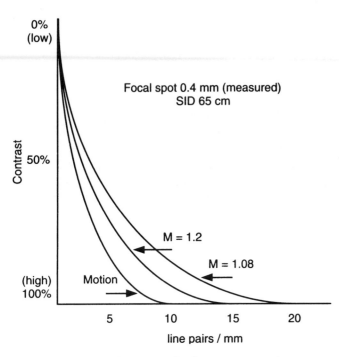

Figure 6.4. Modulation transfer function curves for contact with magnification of M = 1.08 (poorly compressed breast), with magnification M = 1.2, and breast motion.

complex interplay of optical density, resolution, and contrast contributes to the definition of sharpness, which is a perceptual characteristic rather than a quantitative one. A lack of contrast or resolution, or their display within an unsuitable range of optical densities, leads to decreased sharpness.

IMAGE RECEPTOR RESOLUTION

In mammography, image receptor resolution depends on the extent of dispersion of light photons by the intensifying screen transmitted to the adjacent film. The less the dispersion, the greater the resolution. Although film has sufficient resolution to encode whatever imaging information is sent to it by the mammography system, screens can degrade resolution by several factors, all of which will be discussed in Chapter 8. In this chapter we will mention only that screens can degrade resolution, as can poor film-screen contact. Dirt, other artifacts, and noise (quantum mottle) also degrade resolution. These factors will be covered in Chapter 8.

Suggested Readings

Barnes GT, Frey GD. Screen film mammography: imaging considerations and medical physics responsibilities. Madison WI: Medical Physics, 1991:77–100.

    This section gives details concerning anode and tube angles and their effect on focal spot length. How physicists measure focal spots and the allowable tolerances in focal spot size are also discussed technically.

Haus AG. Evaluation of image blur (unsharpness) in medical imaging. Med Radiogr Photog 1985;61: nos. 1 and 2 (also available from Eastman Kodak, Rochester, NY 14650-0801).

    This is a readable, accurate description of modulation transfer function and how it can quantify radiographic resolution.

Selman J. The fundamentals of x-ray and radium physics, 8th ed. Springfield IL: Charles C. Thomas, 1994:205–219.

    A simple description of x-ray tube anodes and cathodes for general radiography.

PROBLEM 1

These magnified views were obtained with different sized focal spots of different mammography units. Why is the upper image so much more detailed than the lower one? Why is the lower image darker (see *arrows*)?

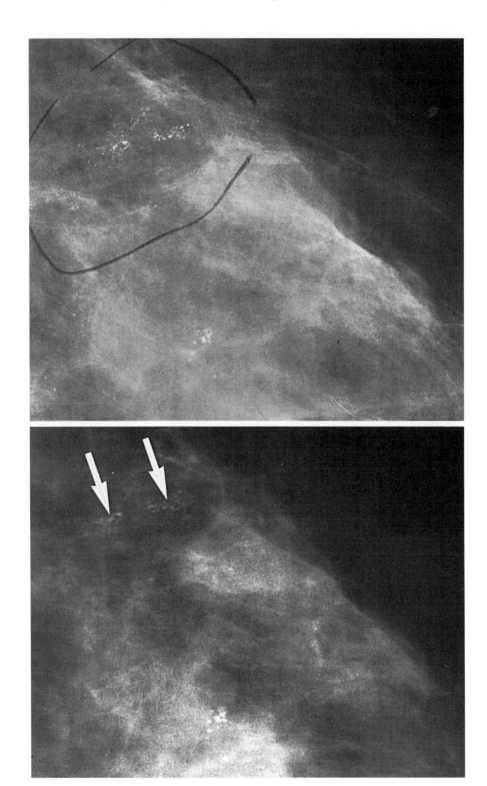

SOLUTION 1

The upper image was produced with a microfocal spot half the size of the lower image. It has less blur and therefore can depict much smaller calcifications. However, mA output is only one-fourth that available for the lower image, so a long exposure was needed to achieve the same film darkening. Such a long exposure was not possible, so the image is lighter than that made with a larger focal spot.

PROBLEM 2

There are several small calcifications (*arrows*) in this detail from a high speed screen/film mammogram. Are the other small dots seen in the image also calcifications?

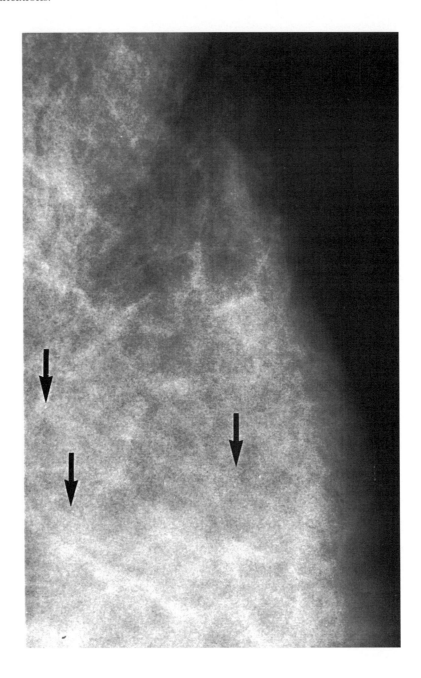

SOLUTION 2

No. The graininess in the image is due to quantum mottle and is the result of a high speed screen/film system and inadequate exposure. Because of such resolution ambiguities, very high speed screen/film systems are no longer recommended by some film manufacturers for screening mammography.

PROBLEM 3

The calcifications (*arrows*) present in this detail are from a mammogram produced by an old mammography unit. The focal spot size was 0.7 × 1.1 mm. Is blurring the only problem in this image?

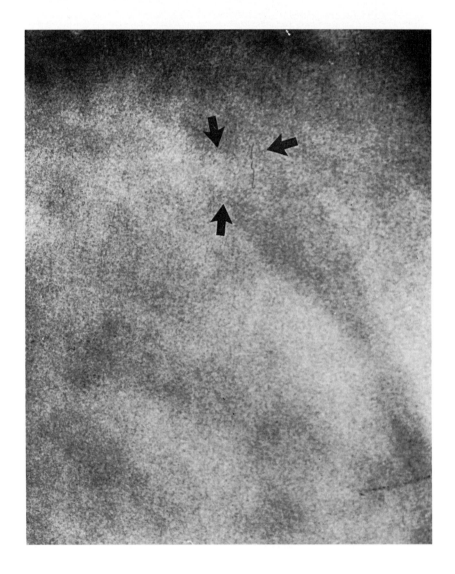

SOLUTION 3

No. Because the unit does not have an antiscatter grid, either reciprocating or fixed, scatter has caused decreased contrast to such an extent that other calcifications are not visible as they are when imaged with a reciprocating grid, below.

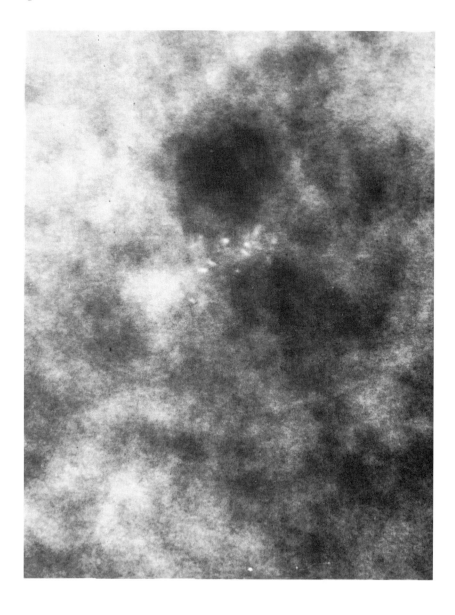

PROBLEM 4

Why are the calcifications in the craniocaudal view so much clearer than the same calcifications in the oblique view (*arrow*)?

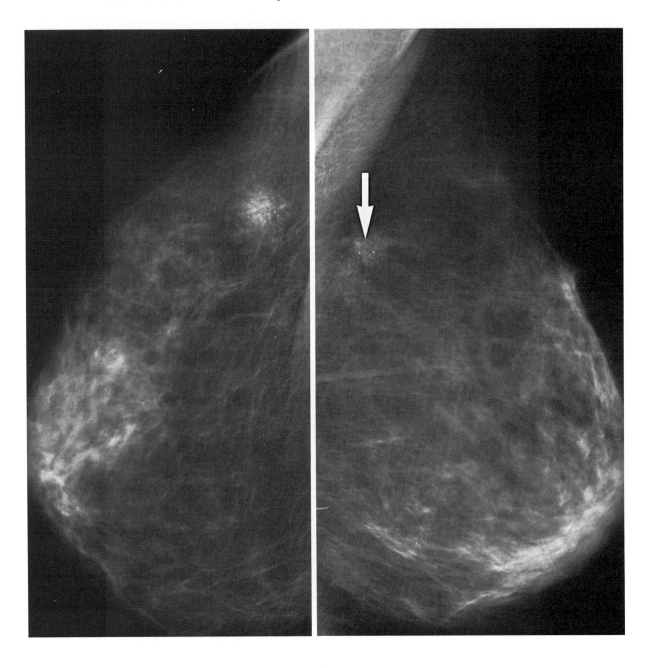

SOLUTION 4

Contrast is the key to this apparent loss of resolution. Because oblique views cannot be compressed as much as craniocaudal views of the same breast, more scatter is generated. Although the film is darker, fewer of the photons represent signal, and most represent noise. The relative position of the object of interest to the film plane also affects resolution. The closer the calcifications are to the image receptor, the less blur will be produced at the edge of each calcification.

PROBLEM 5

Is there a mass (*arrows*) in the mediolateral oblique view or just dense tissue? The craniocaudal view was similarly ambiguous. There is no palpable mass, and ultrasound was also ambiguous. How would you enhance the examination? Would additional views help?

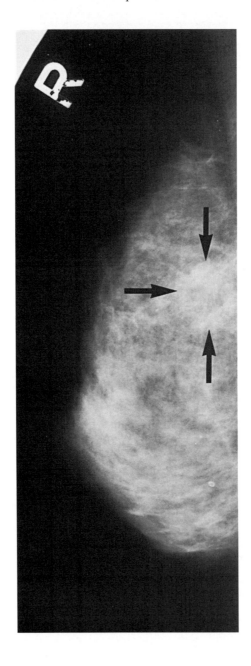

SOLUTION 5

A magnified view shows the edges of the mass clearly. Magnification is helpful for mass detection as well as for clarifying the nature of calcifications. A spot-magnified view was not used because of the large size of the suspicious area and because the mass was not palpable.

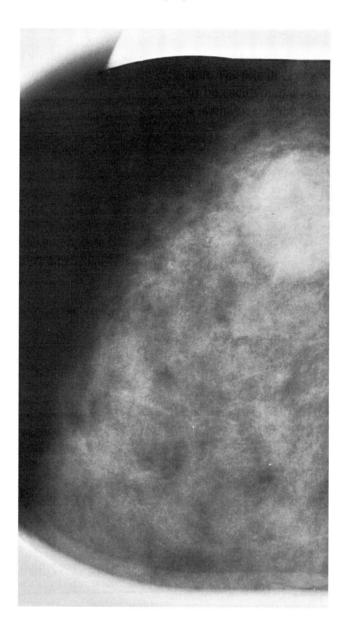

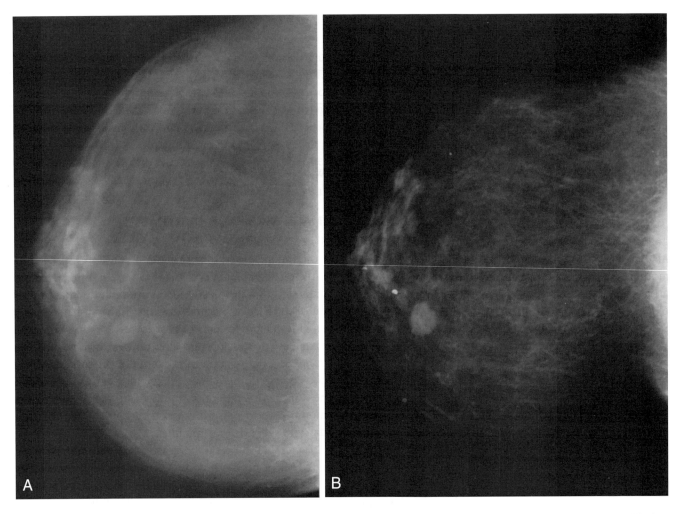

Figure 7.1. **A.** Image was obtained with a W anode unit and aluminum filtration; low contrast film allowed visualization of the skin line. **B.** Image of same breast obtained with a Mo an-ode mammography unit and 0.03-mm Mo filtration. Modern high contrast mammography film shows poor depiction of the skin line.

The difference between attenuation coefficients for different types of breast tissues decreases as kVp increases. Above 40 kVp, film-screen combinations may not be able to show differences among breast tissues owing to the similarity of their attenuation coefficients (Fig. 7.3).

Screen/film systems require preservation of as much subject contrast as possible. This may be achieved by imaging the breast in the energy range that produces the greatest difference in attenuation coefficients. Figure 7.2 illustrates the difference in attenuation between adipose and glandular tissues at the energies used for film-screen mammography. Based on attenuation coefficient differences, contrast is shown to be three times greater at 25 kVp than at 35 kVp.

Although the theoretical advantage of the added contrast that is gained by imaging below 25 kVp seems attractive, more of the x-ray beam is attenuated by the breast at those lower energies. Thus, with their lower energies, the radiation dose is increased. Measurements with a breast phantom show that the dose at 26 kVp is 1.4 times greater than the dose at 28 kVp, if the optical density is the same in both images.

GENERATORS

Several years ago, mammography x-ray generators produced single- or three-phase rectified pulses. Today, all manufacturers use high-frequency generators. The resultant waveform has less low kVp voltage than a 60-cycle rectified waveform. As a result, a lower kVp setting provides the same contrast as that obtained with a 60-cycle rectified unit operated at higher kVp. In general, manu-

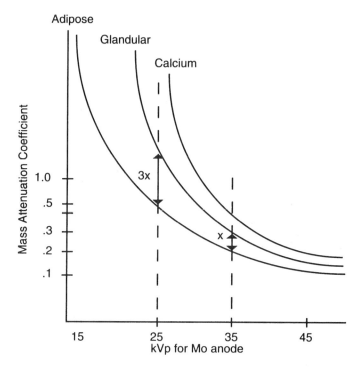

Figure 7.2. Attenuation differences among adipose tissue, glandular tissue, and calcifications can be estimated for each kVp. The graph is an approximation. Note that contrast between adipose and glandular tissue is about three times greater at 25 kVp than it is at 35 kVp.

facturers recommend a reduction of 1–2 kVp to achieve the same contrast as with a 60-cycle rectified unit.

Most high-frequency mammography units use single-phase rather than three-phase generators. During acceptance testing, tube output (mR/mAs) should be tested at the kVp that will be used routinely for imaging average-sized breasts. If 28 kVp was used for an older unit with a three-phase, six-pulse generator and 26 kVp is recommended for optimal contrast with a new high-frequency, single-phase unit, it should be possible to obtain 8 mR/mAs at 26 kVp with the compression plate in place on the high-frequency unit. Excessively long or "timed-out" exposures for large breasts imaged with a grid may force the radiologic technologist to increase kVp to improve tube output, resulting in less subject contrast.

ANODE MATERIALS

Figure 7.1 illustrates the loss of contrast when mammography is performed with a W anode rather than a Mo one. However, some manufacturers now offer mammography units with anodes that have two tracks: one of Mo and a second one of either Rh or W. Because the k-edge for photoelectric absorption of Rh is at 23 keV, and that of W is at 69 keV, the energy spectrum for both

metals is higher than for Mo, whose k-edge is at 20 keV. Mammography units with dual tracks allow the radiologic technologist to select the appropriate energy spectrum for the breast being imaged. One manufacturer suggests that all breasts which cannot be compressed to < 6 cm be imaged with a Rh or W anode. Although this decreases subject contrast, it increases penetration of glandular tissue, which allows small differences in glandular contrast to be recorded at darker optical densities, thus increasing image receptor contrast. Furthermore, calcifications can be better appreciated in a well penetrated mammogram. For large breasts, the savings in dose may be as much as 50% when Rh or W anodes are used instead of Mo.

FILTRATION

If performing mammography with a W anode resulted in the extensive changes in contrast seen in Figure 7.1, few would use this option. In Figure 7.1, note the difference in contrast produced by a W anode and aluminum filtration compared with that produced by a W anode and Rh filtration (Fig. 7.3). The use of a 0.05-mm Rh filter yields an image of a large breast made with a W anode that is almost equivalent in contrast to one made with a Mo anode and Mo filtration. A mammography unit that has only a Mo anode increases its penetration by the substitution of a Rh filter for the Mo filter. The resultant shift in the energy spectrum from 20 keV toward 23 keV not only increases penetration but also reduces mean glandular dose by 15–25%.

In the past, filtration has been mainly used to remove low energy photons from the x-ray beam spectrum. Photons below 15 keV are all absorbed by the breast, and although they contribute to radiation dose, they do not contribute to film exposure. To remove those unwanted low energy x-ray photons, the Mo spectrum x-ray beam is filtered by a very thin (0.03 mm) Mo filter.

Because of the increased attenuation coefficient at low energies, filtration attenuates more low-energy photons than high-energy photons. As a result, the energy spectrum of the beam contains more photons whose energy is closer to the kVp selected (Fig. 7.4). To avoid the excessive filtration that may result from the glass window of an x-ray tube, most mammography x-ray tubes have Be windows. Materials that may inadvertently filter the x-ray beam include an inappropriately positioned mirror for light localization, an excessively thick compression plate, or one made with an inappropriate plastic. All factors that influence filtration can be evaluated by measuring the half value layer of the x-ray beam during acceptance testing the unit.

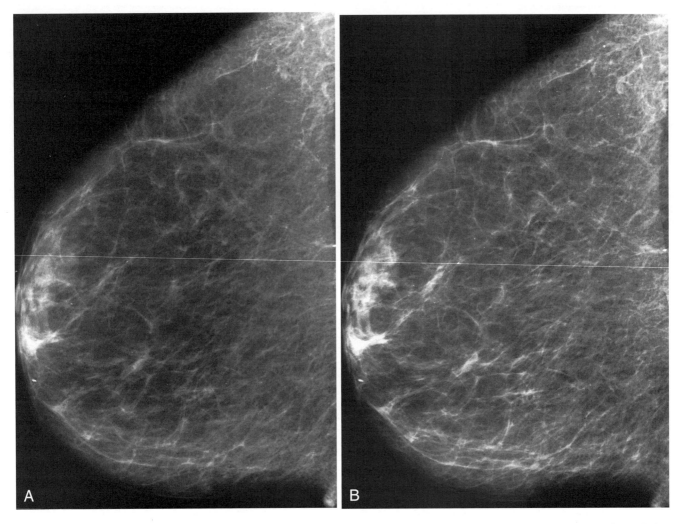

Figure 7.3. **A.** Image was made with a W anode and Rh filter. **B.** Image was made with a Mo anode and Mo filter. Breast remained compressed to a thickness of 6.5 cm for both images.

Finally, some filtration is caused by the breast itself. As x-ray photons traverse the breast, soft, low-energy radiation is attenuated more than higher energy radiation, leading to beam hardening; the greater the thickness of the breast, the more hardened is the beam. Filtration caused by the breast can be measured only by the use of sophisticated procedures and can be minimized by adequate breast compression. Firm compression ranks in importance with appropriate kVp selection as a means of enhancing contrast.

COMPRESSION

Although the role of compression in reducing geometric unsharpness is obvious, its effect on contrast requires explanation. Compression may mistakenly imply to the reader that breast tissue that is 8 × 8 × 8 cm before compression becomes 4 × 8 × 8 cm after compression, so that the same amount of tissue is simply compressed into less space. In actuality, the flattening of the 8 × 8 cm breast tissue also causes it to spread out over a larger area. Because each photon traverses a shorter path of the same atomic mass in the compressed breast, less scatter is generated by that photon, and fewer photons are attenuated. In addition, firm compression reduces the film latitude required to display the image of the whole breast because similar thicknesses of tissue are traversed by each photon, and the overall range of attenuations is decreased. This allows for the use of low latitude, high contrast screen/film receptors, which further enhances contrast. Reduced breast thickness also allows for the use of lower kVp with additional enhancement of contrast.

Spot compression is another method that enhances contrast in a local area of interest (AOI). It has been em-

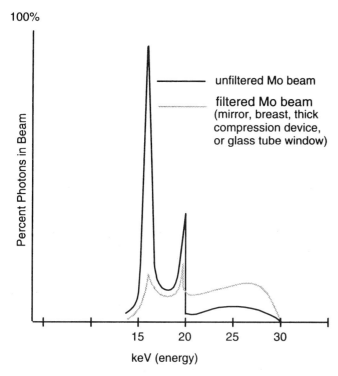

100%

Figure 7.4. Familiar Mo spectrum of a mammography x-ray tube is modified by anything interposed in the x-ray beam. Because x-ray photons at 16 keV are attenuated more than photons at 19 keV, more 16-keV photons are absorbed from the beam. Filtration does not increase the number of 25-keV photons but increases the percentage compared with the total number of photons of all energies left in the beam after filtration.

phasized that spot compression should be used for microfocal magnification images. In fact, a spot compression view may make magnification unnecessary. Combined with magnification, it will result in enhanced contrast and image detail. A small (4- to 6-cm diameter) compression device allows the breast tissue outside the AOI to remain uncompressed, thus permitting tissue in the AOI to be compressed more effectively than with the standard compression device. Contrast is increased by spot compression because fewer low-energy photons are attenuated on their way through the AOI. If the x-ray beam is collimated so that it reaches only the AOI, scatter will be reduced even more and contrast will be further enhanced. Because only the AOI is irradiated, dose to the rest of the breast is minimal.

Small plastic stands that rest on the filmholder and spot-compress the breast from below for craniocaudal views are also available. Because the compression device need not be changed, these stands are preferred for spot compression by some technologists.

GRIDS

Today grids for mammography are of the reciprocating type; i.e., they move during the exposure rather than remaining stationary. The grid moves at the same rate throughout the exposure. Many units initiate movement of the grid as the anode begins rotating, before the exposure commences. Most mammography grids are linear; all are focused for the SID of the unit in which they are installed. The grid ratio, number of grid lines/cm, and interspace material characterize the grid. The grid ratio is defined as the ratio of the height of the grid to the distance between the grid lines. The larger the grid ratio, the more scatter is removed from the image but the greater the additional dose that is required. Grid ratios of 3.5:1 to 5:1 are common in mammography and require a doubling of dose compared with that of a gridless exposure ("Bucky" factor), assuming that the same kVp is used; however, the nongrid technique usually requires 2 kVp less than that with a grid. The number of lines, or lead strips, in the grid will also affect scatter removal and dose. The greater the grid line density, the higher the dose required but the more effective the scatter removal. Mammography grid densities now range from 27 to 46 lines/cm. Mammography grids differ from other radiography grids by having interspaces of carbon fiber rather than aluminum so that the primary photons are only minimally attenuated when they pass through the interspaces. This is important because those photons have already passed through the breast and have contributed to radiation dose.

A recently introduced grid consists of small square cells made of copper. Each cell is focused for the SID of the mammography unit. The interspace material is air. Reciprocation is in one direction, but scatter cleanup is in two directions because the grid cell walls are 45° to the direction of motion.

Innovative moving slots that act as grids for scatter removal are being developed for digital mammography units. They are discussed in Chapter 13.

Of course, no single method for contrast enhancement will suffice unless used with an optimally operating mammography unit, screen/film image receptor, and film processing system.

Suggested Readings

Curry TS, Dowdy JE, Murry RC. Christensen's physics of diagnostic radiology, 4th ed. Philadelphia: Lea & Febiger, 1990:14–17.

This well-known text gives basic information about anodes and filters used in general radiography. This is good background material for understanding how energy spectrums are generated.

Kimme-Smith C, Wong J, DeBruhl N, Basic M, Bassett LW. Mammograms obtained with rhodium vs. molybdenum anodes: contrast and dose differences. AJR 1994;162: 1313–1317.

A study comparing the two anode/filter combinations is described. Radiologists' preferences, mean glandular dose reductions, and type of breast most suitable for the Rh/Rh combination are provided.

Wagner AJ. Contrast and grid performance in mammography. In: Barnes GT, Frey GD, eds. Screen-film mammography: imaging considerations and medical physics responsibilities. Madison WI: Medical Physics Publishing, 1991:115–158.

This technical article, although written for physicists, will also help radiologists and technologists understand the mechanisms of contrast improvement.

PROBLEM 1

These calcifications (marked by a radiopaque O) are thought to be in the skin rather than the parenchyma. How can this be verified without losing contrast at the skin line? (Tangential views might be overexposed at the skin line, possibly preventing visualization of the calcifications.)

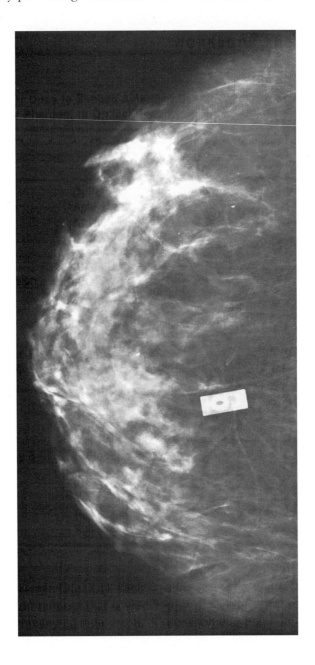

SOLUTION 1

By underexposing the image using manual technique (or −3 on the density setting of the automatic exposure control), the skin retains sufficient contrast to be visible, along with the calcifications (*arrow*) within it.

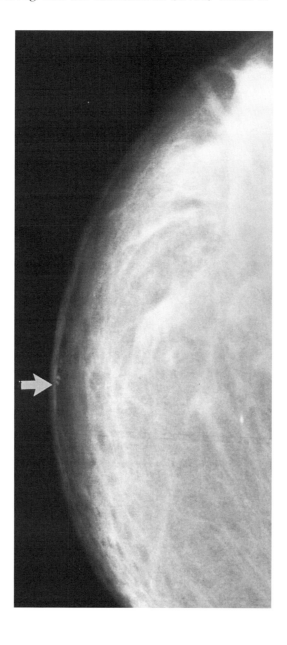

PROBLEM 2

The calcifications in this oblique view are not well characterized and cannot be seen clearly. What view would improve their clarity?

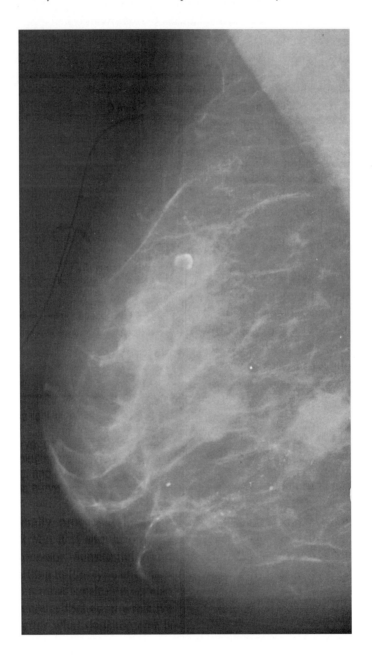

SOLUTION 2

Because less tissue must be penetrated in a craniocaudal view than in a medi-olateral oblique view, it has more contrast and shows the calcifications with greater clarity. They are suspicious for malignancy.

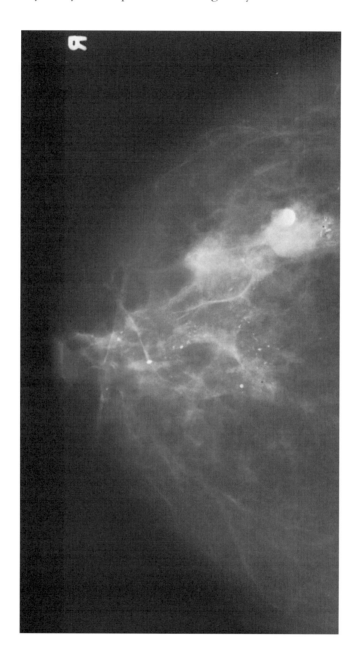

PROBLEM 3

This small (3.5 cm thick) dense breast with a lead marker over a palpable mass is underpenetrated. What can be done to improve the image when the examination is repeated?

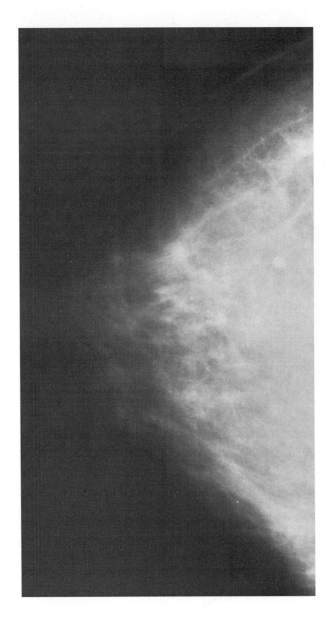

SOLUTION 3

Compression was insufficient, and the automatic exposure control sensor was positioned incorrectly. A repeat examination with proper compression led to good penetration near the chest wall.

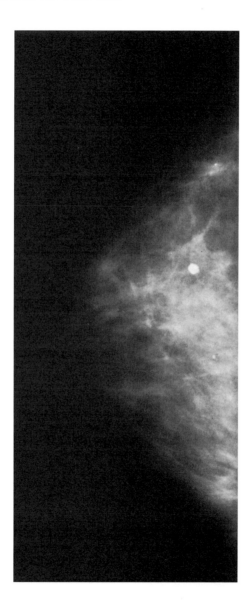

PROBLEM 4

This dense 6-cm-thick breast was imaged at 28 kVp for 3 seconds. The phototimer was set for +1 to give 15% more exposure. What can be done to improve contrast?

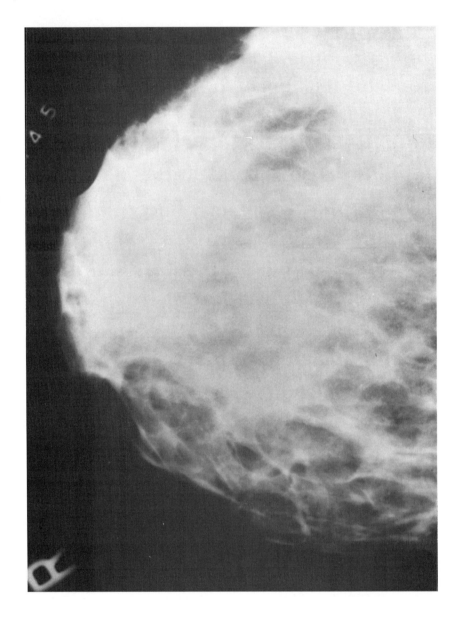

SOLUTION 4

kVp was increased to 30 to increase penetration. This patient would be a good candidate for W/Rh or Rh/Rh imaging. Contrast could be maintained by imaging the breast at 26 kVp with either a W or Rh anode, and mean glandular dose would be reduced 40–55%.

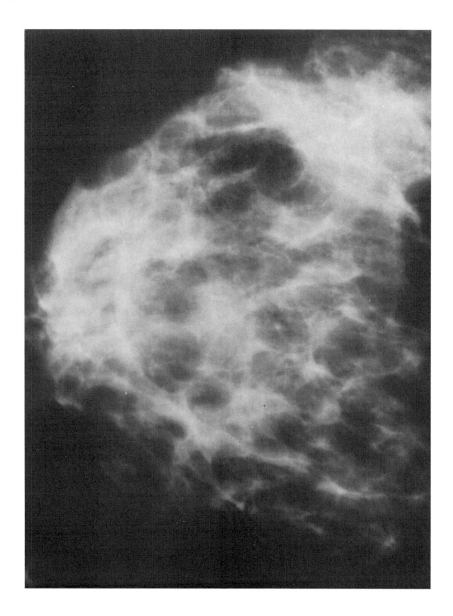

PROBLEM 5

The image on the left was obtained on a modern Rh/Rh mammography unit imaging a very dense 4-cm-thick breast. Her previous films on a Mo/Mo unit (image on right) showed a dense parenchyma but much more detail. Is this an example of the lower contrast expected with a Rh/Rh unit or is there some other problem?

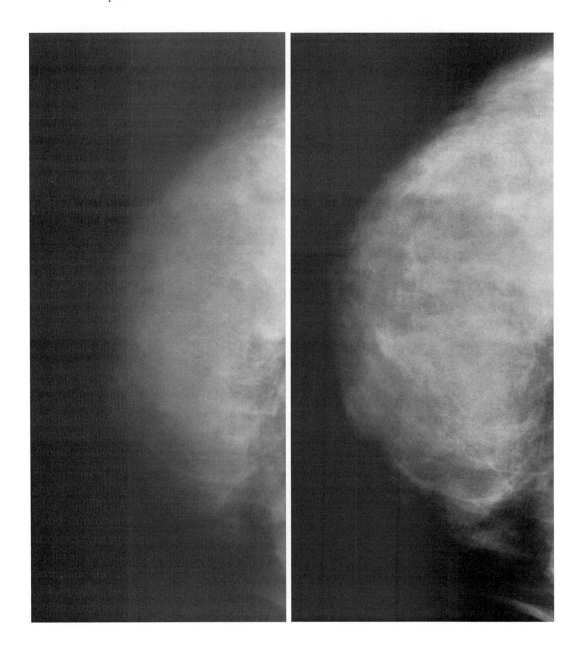

SOLUTION 5

The previous case done in the room containing the Rh/Rh mammography unit required magnification. Because, for magnified views, the grid is replaced with a cassette holder, no grid was present on the unit. When preparing to image this patient, the technologist removed the magnification stand and replaced the compression paddle but forgot to replace the grid. Therefore, the breast was first imaged without a grid. The image below was obtained with a Rh/Rh combination and a grid.

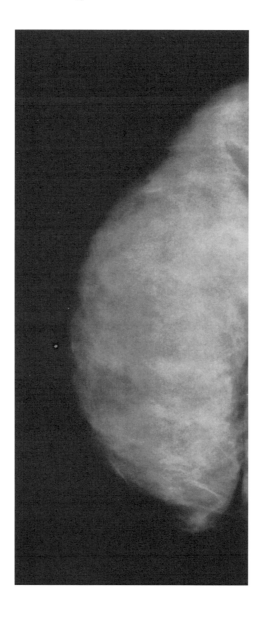

QUESTIONS

1. To avoid using a grid, why can't we image the whole breast with the microfocal spot, using an air gap and large image receptor?

2. A patient who had a recent biopsy cannot tolerate even moderate compression. How can a diagnostic mammogram be performed without hurting her?

3. A radiology center does not have a dedicated high-intensity mammography viewer. What radiological technique could be used to compensate for the contrast that is lost under this suboptimal viewing condition?

4. If a Mo anode/Rh filter improves penetration of glandular tissue, what would a Rh anode/Mo filter do?

5. Why can a cyst that is aspirated and then filled with air be seen in a mammogram when the same cyst was not visible before it was drained?

ANSWERS

1. Most breasts would not fit on a 24 × 30 cm image receptor if they were magnified through the use of a large enough air gap (15 cm) to clean up scatter. Furthermore, because the cathode of the microfocal spot is usually focused on an anode track with a greater angle than the track of the large focal spot (to decrease its size), the field of view is decreased. Finally, if the kVp is kept the same as it would have been for the grid exposure, soft radiation will be attenuated by the air gap more than higher energy radiation, resulting in less contrast. The radiation dose may be higher than when imaging with the grid because of attenuation of photons by the air gap.

2. It is not possible to perform an adequately detailed mammogram. The lack of compression will lead to poor contrast. It would be best to delay imaging for 2 weeks. For a premenopausal patient, the next examination should ideally occur 2–3 days after the onset of the menstrual cycle.

3. The supervising radiologist should be encouraged to correct this deficiency. Shutters can be simulated by providing cardboard or blackened film cutouts of various sizes to reduce ambient light. Reducing the mammogram's optical density to compensate for low intensity viewers will seriously compromise contrast.

4. Because the Rh anode has a k-edge at 23 keV, most beam energy is below that value. A Mo filter filters the energy between 20 and 23 keV, providing a spectrum closer to that of a Mo/Mo combination. Because Rh anode tubes have lower output than Mo anode tubes, it would be more efficient to use a Mo/Mo combination in the first place.

5. Cysts are very close in attenuation to glandular tissue at mammography energies. When they are aspirated and filled with air during a pneumocystogram, contrast is improved because of the difference in attenuation between glandular or adipose tissue and gas.

8

SCREEN/FILM

No single factor in mammography has been more responsible for dose reduction than the screen/film combination. Five years ago, screen/film resolution was so high that geometric resolution could not match it. To reduce the dose to the patient, several film manufacturers increased the speed of their screens, which reduced image receptor resolution and led to severe quantum mottle. During the last 2 years, manufacturers have discouraged breast imagers from using these high speed systems. Instead, the trend has been toward systems that have less noise and sharper detail. Most progress in improving image detail while maintaining low dose has been the result of innovative screen manufacturing.

SCREENS

Most state-of-the-art intensifying screens consist of a rare earth phosphor, terbium activated gadolinium oxysulfide. Recently the DuPont Company has introduced lutetium tantalite screens for mammography. Resolution and speed are affected by the size of the phosphor particle, dye in the particle binder, absorption by the back panel, and thickness of the screen. The dye reduces light diffusion, allowing preservation of resolution even when the phosphor thickness is increased to increase speed. Because the color of the dye controls the part of the light spectrum that is absorbed or enhanced during phosphorescence, dye variations cause some screens to phosphoresce with a slightly different frequency spectrum than others. This leads to variations in speed and contrast between the screens of different manufacturers when combined with the same type film. The reverse may also occur in that variations in speed and contrast may arise when various films, each with its own sensitivity to a different range of the spectrum, are combined with the same screen.

Gadolinium oxysulfide screens emit a yellow-green spectrum when terbium activated, whereas lutetium tantalite screens emit a violet spectrum (410 mm) that can interact directly with silver bromide rather than depending on secondary emissions from dyes in the film.

Screens induce a trade-off between speed and resolution that mainly is affected by the screen thickness and density of the phosphor. All gadolinium oxysulfide screens produce the same conversion efficiency of x-ray photons to light photons. Other factors that distinguish one screen from another (e.g., dye, particle size, and back-screen absorption) decrease the speed gained by increases in the thickness of the phosphor and function only to improve resolution. A thick phosphor layer, compared with a thinner layer, decreases resolution by allowing the light photons generated by a single x-ray photon to travel farther in the phosphor before being absorbed by the phosphor or film. Because light photons are generated in all directions, back-panel absorption reduces this blurring by decreasing the number of light photons that have traveled relatively far from the x-ray photon that generated them. Film manufacturers, such as DuPont, Agfa Matrix, Konica, Kodak, and Fuji, offer mammography screens that vary widely in speed. Because screens can only be tested clinically when they are combined with films, Table 8.1 refers to screen/film combinations rather than to screens alone. Because 3-minute film processing and 90-second film processing are equally common, the data derived from using either processing method are shown. Although there are individual differences in resolution, contrast, and maximum film darkening, these differences are not recorded here because they are influenced by subjective preferences and the phantoms used to evaluate those quantities. Table 8.1 shows the mean glandular dose needed for each screen/film processing method to expose the ACR phantom to an optical density between 1.4 and 1.6 at 25 kVp.

Screens are usually replaced when the coating that protects the phosphor layer is damaged, when the cassette is broken so that it no longer is light tight, or when the sponge supporting the screen, which ensures intimate screen/film contact, loses its resiliency. Because screens are usually replaced every 3–4 years and must be cleaned at least every week, screen artifacts are less common now than they were before Mammography Quality Standards Act regulations were imposed. Screen artifacts can be recognized easily because they occur in the same places on

Table 8.1.
Mean Glandular Dose to Expose American College of Radiology
Mammography Phantom to Optical Density 1.4–1.6 at 25 kVp

Film	Screen	Processing Time (*mrad*)	
		90 seconds	3 minutes
Kodak Min R E	DuPont Microvision	127	78
	Agfa Mammoray	78	50
	Kodak Min R	127	78
	Kodak Min R medium	78	50
	Fuji UM med	78	50
	Fuji UM fine	127	78
Dupont Microvision	DuPont Microvision	98	78
	Agfa Mammoray	63	50
	Kodak Min R	98	78
	Kodak Min R medium	78	50
	Fuji UM med	78	50
	Fuji UM fine	98	63
Fuji Mima	DuPont Microvision	127	78
	Agfa Mammoray	78	50
	Kodak Min R	127	98
	Kodak Min R medium	78	50
	Fuji UM med	78	50
	Fuji UM fine	127	78
Agfa Mammoray 5	DuPont Microvision	127	78
	Agfa Mammoray	78	50
	Kodak Min R	127	98
	Kodak Min R medium	78	63
	Fuji UM med	78	63
	Fuji UM fine	127	98

every film made with a particular screen (Fig. 8.1). Each screen should have an identification number that is visible, but not obtrusive, on the accompanying radiograph. This will allow the screen that causes the artifact to be identified for cleaning or discarding. Information regarding the care and performance testing of screens is provided in Chapter 11.

FILM

Image receptor resolution is limited by the screen, not by the film. Mammography film is single-sided and has greater contrast than general purpose film. Also, the dyes in the film make it responsive to the green light photons produced by terbium-activated rare earth screens. Film that is responsive to green light is called ortho film. Fast film, however, may produce an apparent decrease in resolution because of excessive quantum mottle and a predisposition to processing and handling artifacts that result from greater film sensitivity (Fig. 8.2). Speed and contrast, the two technical parameters usually associated with film, are tested by exposing the film to a graduated amount of green spectrum light (for ortho film) in a sen-

sitometer. The film is then processed in the mammography processor. The resultant gray values are read by a densitometer that converts each gray value to an optical density value. Plotting the optical densities on a graph so that each gray step becomes a value along the *x*-axis produces a characteristic curve for the film (Fig. 8.3). Curves for different films can be compared to determine which film is faster and which has more contrast. Figure 8.4 illustrates the differences between two mammography films. Because film A is closer to the *y*-axis than film B, film A is faster than film B. That is, film A received fewer light photons than film B to obtain the same optical density. Because the straight part of the curve for film B is more vertical than the same portion of the curve for film A, contrast is greater for film B. This implies that a small difference in the number of light photons will result in a larger difference in optical density for film B compared with film A.

Important technical factors inherent in film, other than speed and contrast, are the lowest and highest optical densities that can be represented on the film. If the lowest optical density, the base + fog value, is too high

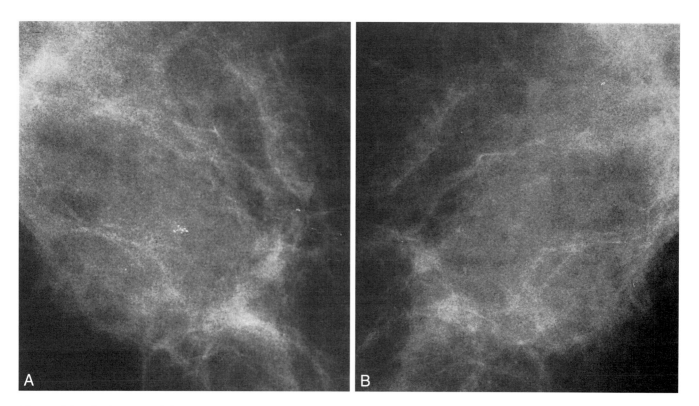

Figure 8.1. **A.** A screen defect masquerades as calcifications. **B.** Same breast imaged with a different screen.

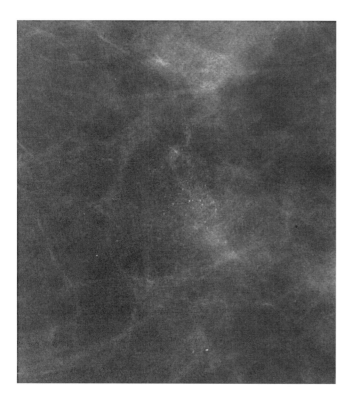

Figure 8.2. Fast mammography film can be damaged by abrasion occurring in the film bin or when the film is gripped too firmly before exposure. The resultant artifact simulates microcalcifications.

(>0.2), then small calcifications (which are likely to have an optical density close to base + fog) will not have as much contrast, compared with glandular tissue, as they would have had on a film with a lower value of base + fog. Similarly, if the maximum gray value (D_{max}) is too low, the skin line may not be visible when "hot-lighted." Contrast that is too high may also prevent the skin from being seen with the aid of a high-intensity light because of excessively decreased latitude.

Another parameter, difficult to measure but easy to see when the characteristic curves of two films are compared, is film gamma at a particular optical density. Even if the average gradient of the characteristic curve is the same, the contrast in the optical density range where most glandular tissue is imaged (0.6–1.5) is more important than the contrast above 1.8. In Figure 8.5, film A has more contrast in the optical density range where it is important to have contrast than film B, although both curves have the same average gradient (measured at the x-points on the characteristic curve).

COMPARISON OF FILMS

Some mammography films are not intended to undergo extended processing (180 seconds/95°F) and therefore should not be processed using this option. For instance,

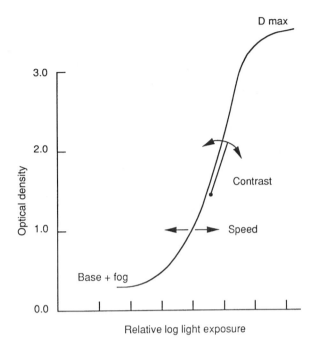

Figure 8.3. Characteristic curve or H & D (Hurter and Drifield) curve that results from plotting optical density versus light intensity. Speed, base + fog, and average gradient (contrast) can be calculated from this curve.

Kodak Min R E is not generally processed in a 90-second processor, and Kodak Min R H should only be processed in a 90-second processor. Sensitometry and densitometry values vary according to film type and manufacturer. The light output from most sensitometers also differs. Because densitometers are calibrated, the relative speed will be accurate no matter what densitometer is used.

Densitometer values obtained from sensitometer strips allow the comparison of different films or the same film from two different manufacturing lots. Although sensitometers are invaluable quality control tools, selection of screen/film combinations based on sensitometric results alone will lead to disappointment. Many other qualities should be considered: price, service, manufacturing stability, processing stability, and the film's sensitivity to abuse before and during processing. Although preliminary selection of screens and films might be based on these qualities and sensitometric results, clinical trials are essential to determine the combination that is most satisfactory for a particular facility (Fig. 8.6). Most manufacturers are willing to lend samples of their screens and to provide film for testing if assured that a sufficient volume will be purchased should the customer decide to buy. Many combinations of films and screens provide similar speed and contrast. Subtle differences in the base

color of the film or in the cassettes provided with the screens may also affect decisions.

Increased film contrast may be necessary if a mammography unit is operated at an excessively high kVp in compensation for a limited mA output. This produces a trade-off of subject contrast for image receptor contrast. Screen/film combinations that are now considered obsolete can be replaced with combinations that require a lower dose for the same resolution.

FILM RECIPROCITY LAW FAILURE

When light photons expose a film, the atoms of silver in each film grain become a latent image center or sensitivity speck to form the nucleus for the development of that grain. About four atoms of silver are necessary for the image center to remain stable until it is developed. If too few atoms of silver are generated in a specified time, the exposed atoms will leave the latent image center, causing that film grain to remain undeveloped. When mammography exposures are long, many exposed film grains may lose their atoms of silver in this way. This process, called "reciprocity law failure," implies that a 0.1-second exposure at 200 mA (20 mAs) will produce a higher optical density than a 1.0-second exposure at 20 mA (also 20 mAs). Different films have different rates of reciprocity law failure. Films can be tested for relative reciprocity law failure with two exposures, at equal kVp

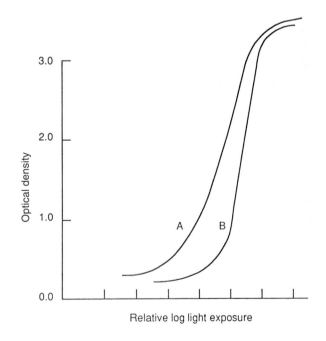

Figure 8.4. Characteristic curves of two films from different manufacturers. Film A is faster than film B, but film B has more contrast than film A.

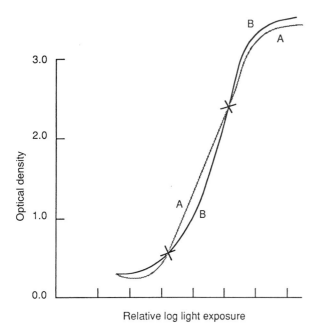

Figure 8.5. Although the average gradients of these two characteristic curves are the same and the speed is only slightly different, film gamma (or contrast) in the optical density range of 0.5–1.5 is superior for film A and will result in greater contrast in glandular tissue.

and mAs, of a phantom: one made with the large focal spot of a calibrated mammography unit and the second made with the microfocal spot of the same unit. The difference in optical density between the two films is the relative reciprocity law failure of the film.

If very long exposures are needed by an underpowered x-ray tube or small focal spot, a film with less reciprocity law failure may be needed to avoid increased dosage to the patient.

LATENT IMAGE FADING

Occasionally, exposed film cannot be processed promptly. The delay in processing may cause some of the sensitivity specks formed by the exposure, and consisting of at least four silver atoms, to recombine with the bromide ions present in the undeveloped film. The process of losing these sensitivity specks is called "latent image fading" and can reduce film optical density 5–20%, depending on the length of time between exposure and processing. Most mammography films do not fade sig-

nificantly (more than 5%) when developed within 8 hours of exposure. However, when processing is delayed 2–3 days, as might occur when a mobile mammography van without an on-board processor serves a remote area or is used on weekends, speed loss of 20% is not unusual. If processing is stable, the latent image fading characteristic of a film can be tested by exposing five film sheets with the ACR phantom at the same manual technique. The first film sheet should be developed immediately and the remaining four sheets at 4 hours, 8 hours, 24 hours, and 48 hours, respectively. Differences between the optical densities of the five films will determine the amount of latent image fading resulting from the various delays in processing.

MANUFACTURERS' QUALITY CONTROL

Film manufacturers constantly readjust their manufacturing parameters. Although mammography film is more closely controlled during its manufacture than any other type of film, the control of film specifications is not always exact. Although manufacturers guarantee against more than a 10% variation from average speed and gradient, this allows for a possible 20% variation between film lots and may require the technologist to change the automatic exposure control setting by one or more density values. A manufacturer's film lot can be identified by the numbers printed on the film box. Before accepting a new lot, compare the new film with the present film by exposing five sheets of each to the sensitometer and processing them together throughout the day.

Gradual differences in contrast are usually detected by the radiologist when comparing previous mammograms to new mammograms. Even when speed and average gradient remain similar, contrast variations near optical density 1.0 can lead to significant clinical differences.

If you encounter visual differences between previous films and new ones, you might compare your evaluation with that of other breast centers who are using the same film. Manufacturing errors often go undetected until customers corroborate poor film performance. Of course, processor variation (see Chapter 9) must be excluded before film variation can be considered the cause of deteriorating image quality.

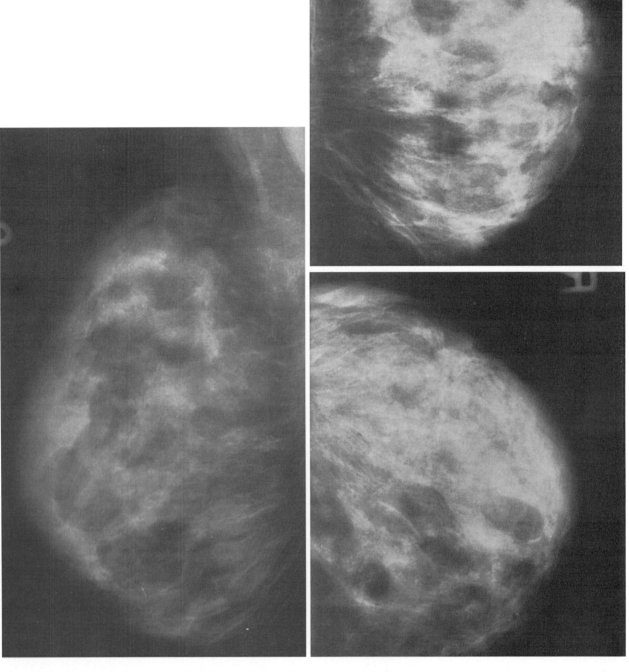

Figure 8.6. These three images resulted from a clinical trial in which three different screen/film cassettes were tested on different breasts and on different views of the same patient.

Suggested Readings

Haus AG. Screen-film image receptors and film processing. In: Haus AG, Yaffe MJ, eds. Syllabus: a categorical course in physics. Technical aspects of breast imaging, 3rd ed. Radiological Society of North America 80th Annual Meeting, Nov 27–Dec 2, 1994.

> This article summarizes the characteristics of mammography screen/film combinations and offers recommendations for their optimal processing.

McKinney WE. Radiographic processing and quality control. Philadelphia: Lippincott, 1988:1–38, 173–198, 215–276.

> While primarily concerned with film development, this textbook describes film storage, cassette and screen maintenance, film manufacturing, sensitometry, film artifacts, and film quality control and provides many helpful and practical suggestions.

Roberts DP, Smith NL, Gunn C. Radiographic imaging, a practical approach, 2nd ed. New York: Churchill Livingstone, 1994.

> Chapters 4 and 5 cover the light spectrum common to medical radiography, the chemistry of film manufacturing, differences in film grain and how speed, contrast, and base + fog are controlled during film manufacture. A similar chapter on screens is equally thorough.

PROBLEM 1

Do the small specks in the image below represent calcifications, screen dirt, or other artifacts?

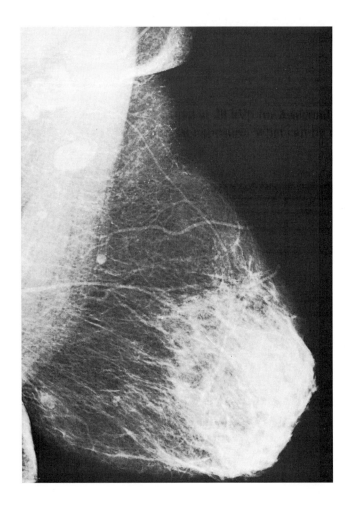

SOLUTION 1

They represent none of these. Note that some of the "calcifications" follow
the contours of the breast and axillary folds. The specks are talcum powder.

PROBLEM 2

What causes the dark line about 1 cm from the chest wall (*arrow*)? All of the films seem to have this artifact.

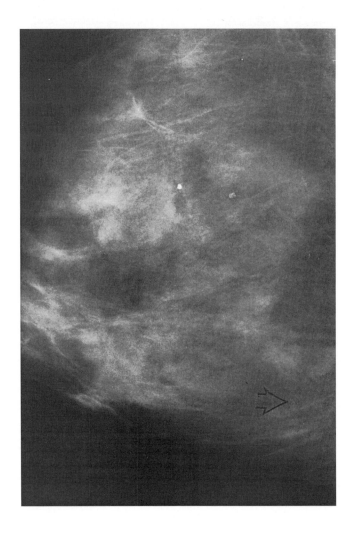

SOLUTION 2

This is the edge of a ridge on the film cassette. When a cassette from a different manufacturer was used, the artifact disappeared.

PROBLEM 3

The image on the left is underexposed, whereas that on the right is correctly exposed. Why can't the cancer in the upper hemisphere be appreciated in the underexposed image?

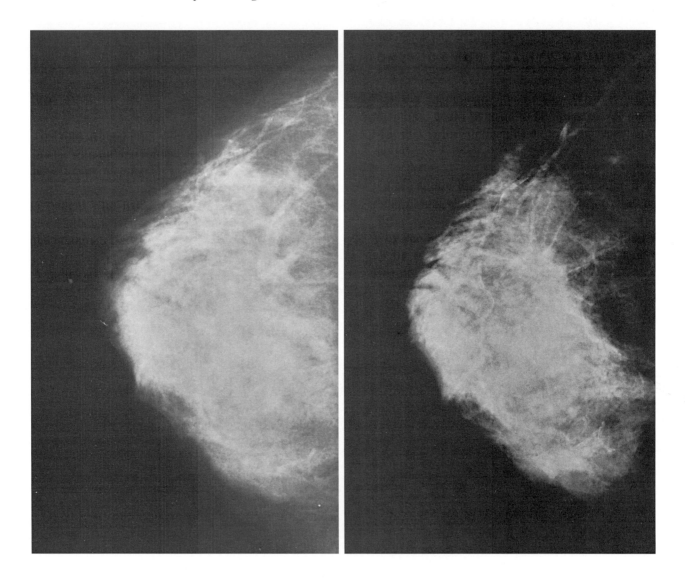

SOLUTION 3

The contrast (gamma) at low optical densities is much lower than at higher optical densities. By moving optical densities on the image up on the film's characteristic curve, contrast is increased.

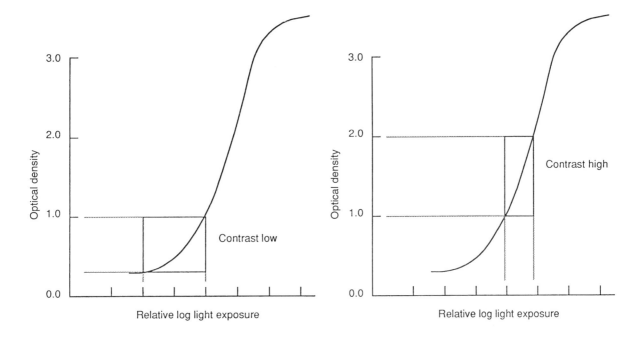

PROBLEM 4

Here, the dark line and the blurring of the image near the chest wall are different than those in Problem 2. Furthermore, they occurred only in this mammogram. What could cause them?

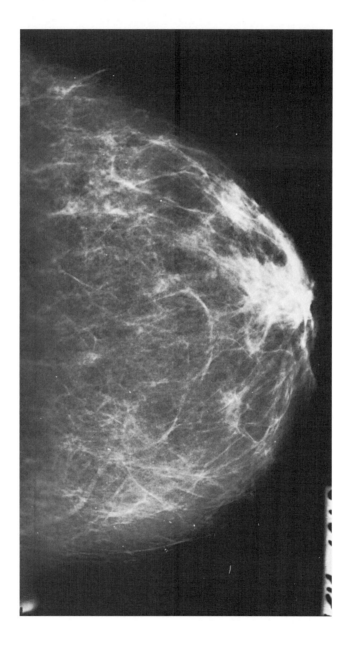

SOLUTION 4

The film was bent, causing the dark line. The blurring was caused by poor screen/film contact owing to the bent film.

PROBLEM 5

Are the calcifications real?

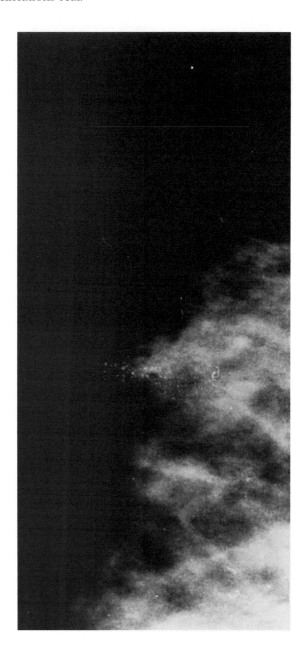

SOLUTION 5

No. Note the other specks of screen dirt on the image. This artifact could also be caused by pick-off, scratches, or other abuse of the screen or film.

QUESTIONS

1. A new box of mammography film was inadvertently exposed to light in the darkroom. However, the film was tightly packed in its box, and, when several sheets in the front and back were processed, only the first and last sheets appeared to have been exposed. Can the rest of the film still be used?

2. The black areas of all the mammograms from one center have a fine pick-off pattern, whereas the sensitometric strips show no such artifact. Is this a screen or a film problem?

3. The text mentions "service" as an attribute of selecting a particular screen/film manufacturer. Beyond taking your film order, what does service entail?

4. The sensitometric values of two different films show that one has an average gradient of 2.6 and the other an average gradient of 2.75. Clinical images made with these films seem to have the same contrast. How is that possible?

5. When testing two screen/film combinations using the same manufacturers' cassettes, a phototimed exposure with one cassette requires twice the mAs compared with the other cassette, but the resulting film is much too dark. Why is this, and how can these two combinations be compared?

ANSWERS

1. No. The top edge of each sheet of film in the box will have been exposed and will be darkened. The base + fog near the exposed edge of each film sheet will be too high. Although the film can be used to adjust the bromide level in the processor (see Chapter 9), it should not be used for imaging.

2. It is a film or processor problem. The sensitometric strips do not show pick-off because they do not contain large areas of exposed film. Excessive pick-off can be a film manufacturing problem. If possible, obtain film from another manufacturer, expose it, and run it through the processor to eliminate the processor as part of the problem.

3. Film manufacturers often provide training programs for radiologists and technologists who use their film. These programs may offer continuing education credits in mammography. The manufacturers have applications specialists who visit a facility and train its technologists in positioning, Mammography Quality Standards Act regulations, and other aspects of mammography quality. Account representatives will help solve processing problems, will intercede with firms servicing your processor, and will replace film that is found to be out of tolerance. Find out how active the film representative is in your geographic area before selecting a particular brand of mammography film.

4. The sensitometer light output simulates the spectrum of light emitted by the screen. The difference between the spectrum of the screen output compared with that of the sensitometer would affect film speed but not have significant contrast effects. Differences in clinical contrast depend on many factors and are difficult to evaluate unless technical factors are carefully controlled. Therefore, the small difference in sensitometrically measured average gradient is unlikely to represent a significant difference in clinical images.

5. The automatic exposure control has been calibrated for one screen/film cassette combination. When a different cassette with a thicker screen or more attenuating backing is introduced, the calibration must be repeated. To compare two screen/film combinations in different cassettes, image the same phantom at the same kVp using a manual technique. Adjust the technique until the optical densities match within 10%. The extent of mAs that is required can be used to help the service engineer recalibrate the automatic exposure control when a decision concerning the screen/film combination has been made. Some mammography units can support the use of two different screen/film combinations, each calibrated to its own range of exposures.

9
FILM PROCESSING

Should the quality of mammography become substandard, the most likely source of the problem is faulty film processing. The chemicals in the film processor undergo change more frequently than the changes that occur in the mammography unit as a result of mechanical or electronic failure. In addition to the problems introduced by the need to periodically replenish or completely replace the chemical solutions, progressive wear and tear over 10 years or more can produce film artifacts that may interfere with diagnostic capability. Although problems in film processing are just as prevalent in other branches of radiology, the exceedingly fast film required for mammography is particularly vulnerable.

FILM DEVELOPMENT PROCESS: FILM FACTORS

Film consists of a plastic sheet coated with a thin emulsion of AgBr grains suspended in gelatin. Contrast depends on the variation in size of the film grains. The more varied the size of the grains, the greater the film latitude and the lower the contrast. Film speed also depends on grain size as well as on the distribution and thickness of the emulsion. During the reduction process, electrons are supplied to the grains that have been exposed to light or x-rays but not to the unexposed grains. Each exposed grain has a latent image center or sensitivity spot that contains at least four atoms of silver. Development amplifies these atoms by reducing all the silver halide in the grain to metallic silver. Raising the temperature of the development solution accelerates the process. The thickness of the emulsion and the shape of the film grains determine the length of time needed for the complete development of the exposed grains to occur. Because flat grains do not require as much time for development as cubic or irregularly shaped grains, several types of mammography film have been manufactured with flat grains, obviating the need for extended processing to obtain complete development. Furthermore, if both sides of the film are coated with emulsion, each coat is thinner than that used in a standard, single-coated film. This also precludes the need for long development time.

Other differences in film that affect development outcome are related to "latent image fading." Some films lose silver atoms from exposed latent image centers more readily than others. Speed reductions of more than 5% may occur when the development of exposed film is delayed for more than 8 hours. Because radiographs performed in a mobile van without an on-board film processor are those most likely to be affected by latent image fading, their processing must not be unnecessarily delayed.

In addition to its usefulness in film quality control, sensitometric exposure of a standard film is also used to measure the performance of the film processor. The only difference in the two quality control procedures is that each periodic evaluation of a processor must be performed with a standard film taken from the same manufacturing lot. This ensures that processor variations rather than film variations are tested. Sensitometric films should be run daily, after any change in processor chemistry and after the processor is repaired. Of course, the sensitometer must be set to match the color spectrum appropriate for the test film. Processor tests to evaluate the chemistry of the developer and fixer are described under "Chemistry."

CHEMISTRY

Two mixtures of chemicals are used for film processing: one that constitutes the developer and the other the fixer. The developer changes AgBr grains to silver, and the fixer stops the development process and washes out the undeveloped silver halide crystals, leaving transparent the unexposed portions of the film. Of the two mixtures, the developer is the most expensive and complex.

The developer contains hydroquinone and phenidone, which function as sources of electrons to reduce the film grains to metallic silver. Hydroquinone controls the contrast and blackness of the fully exposed portions of the film. Because hydroquinone is slow to react fully with the film, its chemical reaction is enhanced by extended processing. Phenidone reacts more quickly and controls speed, particularly in the low optical density areas of the film. The combination of the two organic agents results in greater film speed than either could produce alone. Various other chemical agents are used to protect the developing agents against oxidation, preserve pH balance, swell the emulsion to accelerate development, reduce fog, and moderate the activity of fresh developer.

The alkalinity of the developer is important. Activity can be increased by adding an alkali, or accelerator, to the developer. Because the accelerator causes unexposed as well as exposed film grains to be developed, it is controlled by a restrainer, usually potassium bromide, which is added initially as a "starter" to newly replaced developer. During film development, bromide from the reduced AgBr grains is washed off the film and slows development even more. In fact, the decrease in the activity of the developer is related primarily to the buildup of bromides within it. Testing the alkalinity of the developer assesses its activity and indicates whether its replenishment is sufficient to develop all exposed grains in the film. In the absence of a starter, the developer pH is 10.25 and its specific gravity is between 1.08 and 1.085; when the appropriate amount of starter is added, the pH is lowered to 10.2, and the specific gravity ranges from 1.08 to 1.09. These values, along with others for seasoned developer, are listed in Table 9.1.

Although the pH is easily measured by a technologist with the appropriate paper-strip reagents (which differ for alkaline and acid solutions), the measurement of specific gravity requires a glass hydrometer and a graduated beaker. The solutions must be at room temperature when measured. The measurements are usually made by a technician trained in chemistry or by a physicist. If the chemical solutions are suspected of being too dilute or poorly mixed, the discovery of a decrease in specific gravity will substantiate these suspicions. If the supplier has simply increased the proportion of phenidone in relation to hydroquinone to increase profit (the latter is more expensive to produce than the former), the specific gravity will not be altered.

Because of its alkalinity, the developer is rapidly oxidized by air and gradually turns from its original yellow to brown. Brown developer signifies that it needs replacement. The oxidation of the developer may be slowed by adding a preservative, such as sodium sulfite, to it. Over time, as more bromide from the reduced AgBr grains enters the developer solution, its chemical agents gradually become less active. To maintain a constant rate of development, chemical replenishment is needed. Older processors automatically measure the linear feet of film fed through them and replenish both developer and fixer accordingly. Because the bromides in the film emulsion are dissolved in proportion to the area of the film rather than its linear dimension, factors such as film orientation, the frequency with which two films are fed simultaneously (side by side) into the processor, and film transport speed all affect the rate of replenishment. As a result, many of the more recently designed processors measure film area rather than length, replenishing the solutions accordingly. Film manufacturers recommend that the volume of replenishment should be between 400 and 500 ml for each square meter of film (70 ml per 14 × 17 inch film). For high volume breast imaging centers (more than 30 patients/day), replenishment rates as low as 20 ml/14 × 17 inch film do not affect contrast, base + fog,

Table 9.1.
Typical Developer and Fixer Solution Parameter

	Specific Gravity	pH	Replenishment Rate
Developer solution (with starter) seasoned	1.08–1.1	10.1–10.2	
Developer replenishment solution (without starter)	1.07–1.085	10.25	50–80 ml/35 cm film travel[a]
Fixer solution	1.080–1.130	3.90–4.5	
Fixer replenishment solution	1.080–1.110	3.90–4.20	70–100 ml/35 cm film travel[a]

[a]Recommended replenishment rates depend on the volume of film processed and are for tank processors.

or speed. For imaging centers with low volumes (fewer than six patients/day), "flood replenishment" may be needed to maintain stable sensitometric values.

Some film processors now have computerized replenishment programs by means of which, unless film volume is extremely high (200 films/day), flood replenishment will occur automatically. After weekends, or if processing has not occurred for 8 hours, flood replenishment takes place. This may cause over-replenishment, leading to fluctuations in the speed sensitometric index. Modification of the program controlling replenishment requires a cooperative relationship between the chemical supplier and film processor service person. Because of the high cost of developer, the promotion of unnecessary over-replenishment is all too common and may spur some negotiation to control it.

The fixing solution (fixer) stops the development process and dissolves the unreduced silver halide grains. The fixer contains a solution of acetic acid, which lowers pH and stops development, and ammonium thiosulfate, which reacts with the unreduced AgBr grains to form soluble silver thiosulfate and bromide ions. It also contains a preservative, e.g., sodium sulfite, and water that serves as a solvent. The specific gravity of the fixer ranges from 1.077 to 1.130, and the pH is usually near 4.2. The fixer should have a strong odor of vinegar. Contamination of the developer with fixer causes an ammonia-like odor. The fixer must be replenished periodically because of the build-up of silver thiosulfate and bromide that occurs within it and because residual developer trapped in the film emulsion contaminates the fixer tank and neutralizes the pH of the fixer. Usually the fixer is replenished at a slightly higher rate than that of the developer. A silver recovery system may be attached to the fixer tank. Typical parameters for the fixer replenishment solutions are listed in Table 9.1.

A simple test of fixer activity is called the "clearance test." The test can be performed in daylight and requires 8 ounces of fixer in a pan or dish in which is dipped a corner of a sheet of undeveloped film. Once the film has been submerged in the fixer, it should change from milky to transparent in less than 10 seconds. Failure of the film to change in the allotted time implies that the fixer is no longer active.

High-volume general radiographic processors usually use 90-second processing (including 22 seconds immersion in the developer solution) and a 95°F (35°C) developer temperature. Small-volume (desktop) processors may use a lower temperature [(e.g., 92°F (33.3°C)] to reduce developer oxidation and a longer processing cycle (e.g., 127 seconds) to achieve the same photographic ef-

fect. "Push processing," a method of film development that has long been used by photographers to increase film speed, has become popular in mammography. By increasing the development time and temperature, the film speed can be increased (Fig. 9.1). Increasing the developer temperature results in increased oxidation and is generally not advisable except in high-volume applications. Extending the processing cycle or developer immersion time increases film speed without producing oxidation and therefore is preferable. The thicker emulsion of single-emulsion film may not be developed completely by the conventional 22 seconds of immersion in the developer solution. By doubling the immersion time, the speed of some films may be increased by 35%. For the fine grain emulsions used in mammography, contrast is also enhanced because of the increased hydroquinone reaction, particularly if the temperature during development is between 95°F (35°C) and 98°F (36.6°C). A temperature above this level may increase base + fog and, as previously noted, results in increased oxidation of the developer chemistry.

The frequency of chemistry change depends on whether a mammography facility uses a film processor dedicated entirely to mammography or has to share it. Compared with processing only mammography film, processing a wide variety of film sizes and types has a greater effect on the developer replenishment rate and leads to greater contamination by residual chemicals, necessitating more frequent chemistry changes. A dedicated processor, run at 35°C with a volume of 80–200 films a day, usually needs cleaning and chemistry change no more than every 3–4 weeks. The processor should be turned off at night so that its chemicals can cool. To minimize oxidation, the automixers or replenishment tanks should have lids with undersurfaces that remain in contact with the chemicals. Mammography Quality Standards Act requires that daily sensitometric values are within specified limits. The need to replace chemicals is signified either by an increase in base + fog and a decrease in contrast in the characteristic curve or a decrease in overall speed. Other processor quality control procedures are described under "Processors."

PROCESSORS

Two types of processors are available: a small (2 × 3 × 2 feet) inexpensive desktop processor that has troughs of chemicals and a high replenishment rate and a large (3 × 3 × 5 feet) stand-alone processor in which development chemicals are contained in a tank (Fig. 9.2).

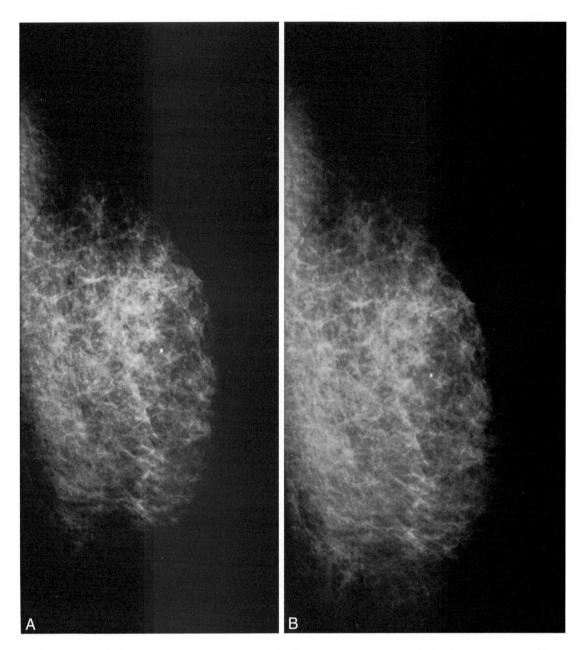

Figure 9.1. Both mammograms were exposed with the same technique. **A.** 3-minute processor. **B.** Same processor but developed for 90 seconds.

"Straight-through" desktop processors require carefully adjusted replenishment rates to maintain their small volume of chemicals. Small errors can cause large imbalances in chemistry, resulting in an instability of speed and contrast that may be particularly marked in extended cycle processing. Moreover, should the developer not be sprayed evenly on the film, irregularities in optical density may result. Small processors have certain advantages in addition to their cost and compact design. Because the film travels in a straight line, it is handled by fewer rollers and is less subject to roller artifacts. In addition,

because development can occupy two of its four stations, extended processing can be implemented in less than 3 minutes. Fresh chemicals are washed over each film so that oxidized chemicals are less likely to decrease speed and contrast. Infrared drying also reduces roller artifacts.

Both types of processors require water to wash the fixer from the film. Although some purists have suggested that softened water performs this task better than hard water, most municipal water supplies are sufficiently free of dissolved minerals to rinse the film adequately. Nevertheless, all incoming water pipes should be fitted

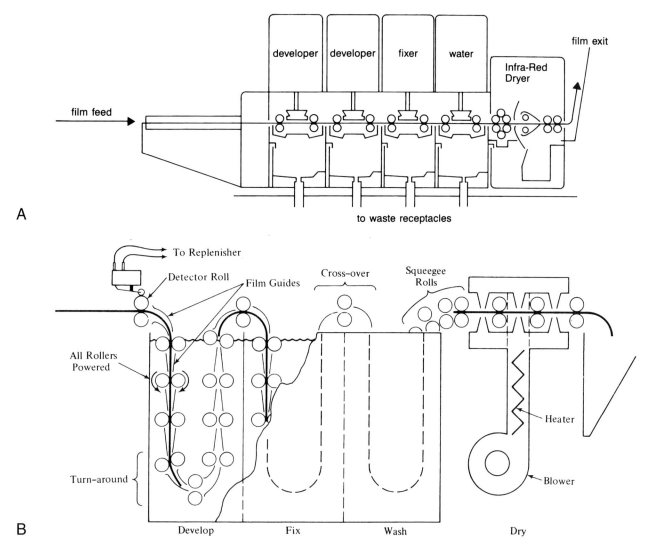

Figure 9.2. Two types of processors are available. A desk-top-sized processor (*top*), in which fresh chemicals wash over the film as it travels through the processor and then the film is dried by the heat of lamps. Compare this processor with the tank type processor (*bottom*), in which complex, paired rollers transport the film through tanks of agitated chemicals, finally to be dried by a hot-air blower.

with a 40- to 50-micron filter to dispose of particulate matter that might otherwise scratch the soft film emulsion. Although some processor maintenance firms recommend filters as fine as 20 microns, these must be replaced more frequently than 50-micron filters. Should particulate matter clog the filter, the flow of rinse water will decrease, resulting in the retention of fixer on the films.

Tank-type processors also agitate the chemicals, increasing the supply of fresh chemicals that come into contact with the film grains. Should the recirculation pumps cease to function properly, the film is likely to be unevenly developed because some chemicals will remain on parts of the film longer than on other parts of the film and because the temperature varies in the development tank.

The film rollers consist of four types: crossover, guide, turnaround, and squeegee. The crossover rollers carry the film from the developer to the fixer and from the fixer to the water tanks. They gently squeeze as much of the chemicals out of the film as possible. During this process, they also squeeze the chemicals into the film emulsion, aiding development or fixation. Too much roller pressure causes marks to appear in the softened film emulsion, and too little pressure results in the film carrying an excessive amount of developer into the fixer tank, wasting the developer and deactivating some of the acetic acid in the fixer. Because the guide rollers carry the film into and out of the tank, their speed must be coordinated throughout all the tanks. Turnaround rollers are a main source of the artifacts that occur when the film scrapes the bottom of the tank. They are also the most likely culprits if a roller misadjustment causes the film to jam. This is because a film that fails to turn around in the tank will interfere with the progress of the films behind it. Squeegee rollers prepare the film for drying. Again, artifacts can result from irregularities on the roller surfaces caused by dirt or contamination.

Film drying seems like a simple process, but associated mishaps can adversely affect film quality. The most obvious is incomplete drying of the film; when stored in a film jacket, the still soft gelatin of the emulsion will adhere to adjacent film surfaces, ruining them. If the interior of the processor (outside the tanks) is not kept free of dust and dried, spilled chemicals, the blower will transfer this foreign material onto the still soft film emulsion, leaving artifacts. If the hot air heater does not shut off during the time between the processing of one film and the next, the processing chemicals may overheat, causing increases in film fog and speed and a decrease in contrast.

AUTOMATIC LOADERS (DAYLIGHT SYSTEMS)

Some film processors can now be fitted with a cassette loader and unloader which feeds exposed film sheets directly into the processor. In the darkroom, unexposed sheets of film are transferred from the manufacturer's box to a lightproof canister. The canister is placed in an automatic loader to which special cassettes are matched. For some mammography x-ray units, the tunnel that houses the film cassette will have to be modified to securely hold the special cassettes, which are thinner than the usual cassettes. These special cassettes may have markers on both their outside and inside to enable the automatic equipment to recognize the orientation of the cassette.

Besides the obvious advantage of increased throughput, automatic loaders have three other advantages:

1. They decrease film handling artifacts and reduce the frequency with which screens must be cleaned.
2. If the facility has a mobile mammography van without a processor, thus necessitating batch processing, the exposed films can be placed in a special canister and processed automatically at the main facility.
3. The number of films developed per day is automatically recorded by the automatic loader and is available to the user.

However, a darkroom is still needed in which to carry out daily quality control tests and load the canisters with unexposed film. Because the daylight loader's automatic film handling mechanism may occasionally jam, an alternate conventional processor, sensitometrically matched to the one servicing the automatic loader, should be available for use when needed. Occasionally, film handling artifacts can be seen in films developed in a daylight system (Fig. 9.3).

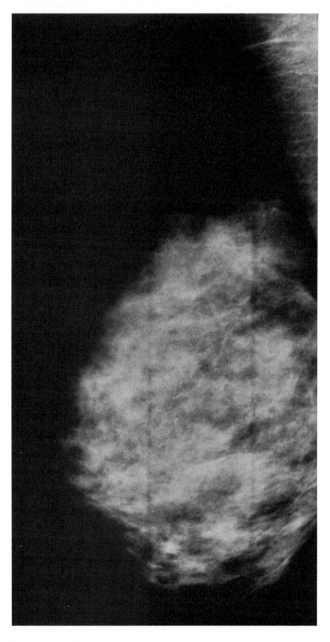

Figure 9.3. "Fingers" in the automatic loading processor may leave regularly spaced streaks on the film when their pressure is too great.

PROCESSOR MAINTENANCE

Processor maintenance consists of many procedures, most of which tend not to be performed rigorously enough. Processors are usually repaired only when they become inoperable, leading to loss of the use of the radiology facility for several hours and, possibly, for days. To avoid processor breakdown, proper maintenance is essential.

After the last radiographs of the day have been processed, the technologist should turn off the processor, drain the water from the rinse tank, and remove the crossover rollers and rinse them with fresh water. Some processors now drain the water automatically once they are turned off. The processor lid should be replaced but left slightly ajar to allow the processor to cool rapidly. The lid prevents the entry of grit from ceiling ventilators. Whenever chemicals are changed, the tanks should be rinsed, drained again, and wiped dry to remove any solid matter that might adhere to films. Developer filters and water filters should be changed routinely, not merely when they appear dirty. Every month, the thermostat should be checked against an independently calibrated metal or digital medical thermometer (never a mercury thermometer!). Every 3 months, the side panels of the processor should be removed to allow inspection of hoses and hose clamps. Because most control electronics, pump motors, and thermostats are located at the bottom of the processor, they are easily damaged by fluid leaking from hoses. Careful periodic inspections will spot worn hoses before they leak and will foster timely replacement.

Roller damage can be detected by exposing mammography film to small amounts of radiation and then developing these "flood films," feeding them into the processor in various orientations. A sheet of plastic 0.5 inches to 2 cm thick will probably be required to act as an attenuator during a manual exposure. An optical density between 1.1 and 1.4 is optimal for these tests. At least four films will be needed. Two should be fed into the processor emulsion side down and two emulsion side up. Each pair should be fed into the processor in different orientations: e.g., the first film long edge first and the next short edge first. If films are usually fed into the processor lined up with either the right- or left-hand film guide, then four more films should be processed using the right-hand film guide if the left-hand guide was already used or vice versa. The processed flood films should not have streaks or scratches in the direction of or perpendicular to the direction of their travel through

the processor. Streaks perpendicular to the direction of travel are symptoms of binding or excess roller pressure. Scratches in the direction of travel are the result of dirt on the rollers (Fig. 9.4). If the film that was fed emulsion side down is scratched, the turnaround boots at the bottom of the tanks may need to be adjusted. Rollers should never be soaked in a cleaning solution because they will absorb it, and the retained solution in the rollers may affect the processing chemistry. Instead, the rollers should be wiped down, scrubbed, and then thoroughly rinsed.

Although developer replenishment rates can be measured with a "J" tube, they are not routinely measured. A change in the replenishment rate requires measurement by a trained processor technician or physicist. A J-shaped tube inserted into the replenishment input open-

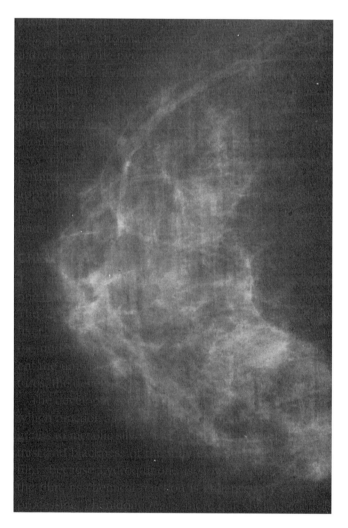

Figure 9.4. Dark streaks are the result of dirt on the rollers causing uneven pressure on the film.

ing allows the replenishment chemical to be collected in a graduated beaker. The amount of replenishment chemical delivered when a film is fed into the processor then can be measured easily.

Some processors come with graduated beakers that can be filled with the fluid expelled during developer replenishment. By measuring this volume, the rate of replenishment can be estimated. However, it may be necessary to obtain measurements during the development of 10–20 films because many modern processors do not replenish the developer after each film is developed. Accidentally exposed films can be used for this calibration.

This chapter concludes the description of the separate components of mammography quality. Chapter 10 concerns radiation dose, particularly its measurement and control.

Suggested Readings

Haus AG. Film processing in medical imaging. Madison WI: Medical Physics, 1993.

A collection of useful papers concerning all aspects of processing. Experts suggest ways to maintain good processing. They describe the chemistry of the development process and analyze artifacts; they explain how to meet Occupational Safety and Health Administration requirements when designing processor facilities and how to cope with processor service persons.

McKinney WE. Radiographic processing and quality control. Philadelphia: Lippincott, 1988.

This is a superb reference for every radiology practice. It is readable, contains practical suggestions, and gives troubleshooting guides for diagnosing a processor's ailment when it develops specific symptoms.

Roberts DP, Smith NL, Gunn C. Radiographic imaging, a practical approach, 2nd ed. New York: Churchill Livingstone, 1994:Chapters 6 and 7.

This is our favorite text for all the chemical details of film processing.

Sprawls P, Kitts EL. Optimum processing of mammographic film. RadioGraphics 1996;16:349–354.

An excellent review of sensitometric methods of processor control and the effects that can occur from processor malfunction and poor chemistry.

PROBLEM 1

Can you find the roller marks? The film was fed into the processor in the orientation shown below. What has caused the marks?

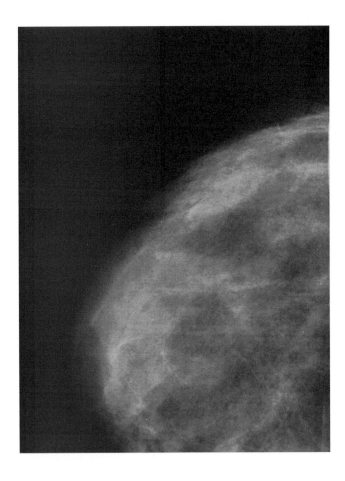

SOLUTION 1

Because the light horizontal lines just above the nipple are oriented in the same direction as the rollers, the rollers must be compressing the film unevenly or are vibrating (chattering) as they rotate. The irregular pressure produces the horizontal lines, which represent insufficient penetration of the developer to the film emulsion.

PROBLEM 2

What are the dark marks on this film?

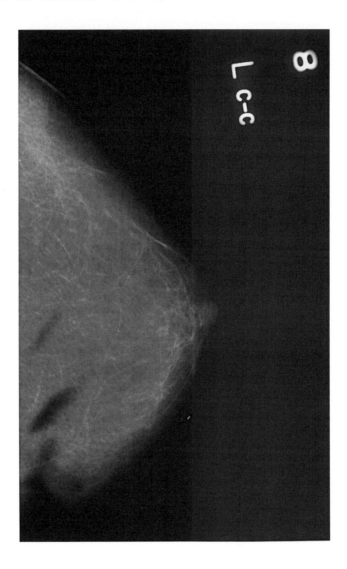

SOLUTION 2

Film fog. Because of their irregular shape, they most likely result from exposure of the film to light in the darkroom (possibly in the film drawer) before being loaded into a cassette and exposed with x-rays. Film that is fogged in the processor usually has a uniformly higher optical density over a rectangular portion of the film.

WORKBOOK FOR QUALITY MAMMOGRAPHY

PROBLEM 3

These two images of an anthropomorphic breast phantom were made at 26 kVp and 40 mAs using the same screen/film combination. The films were developed in different processors at the same facility. What might account for the differences between them? With permission from Radiographics (1992) 12:1145.

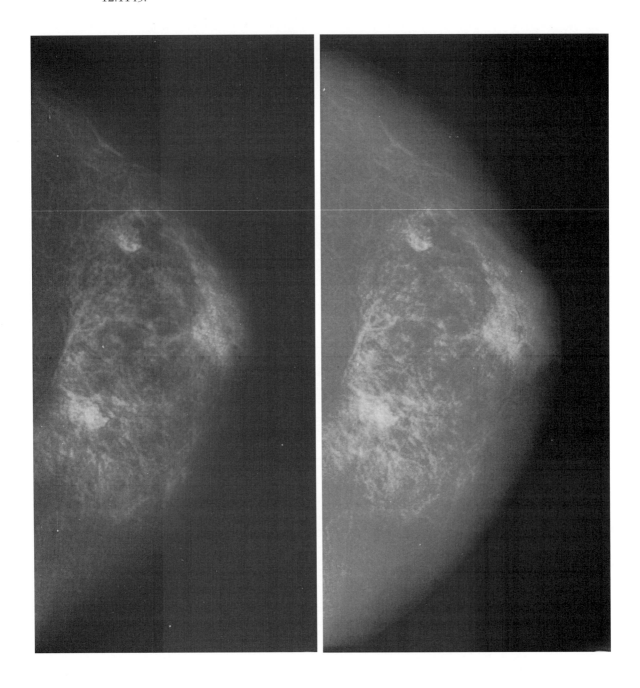

SOLUTION 3

The processing temperature might have been different, with a lower temperature accounting for lower speed and a lighter image. Contaminated developer might also account for the lower speed. If only one processor was used exclusively for mammography, the image with the lower optical density was more likely developed in the nondedicated processor, which may not have been cleaned as frequently as the dedicated processor. The difference in optical density is too great to be the result of a difference in processing speeds.

PROBLEM 4

Do these artifacts represent dirt on the screen or are they processor related?

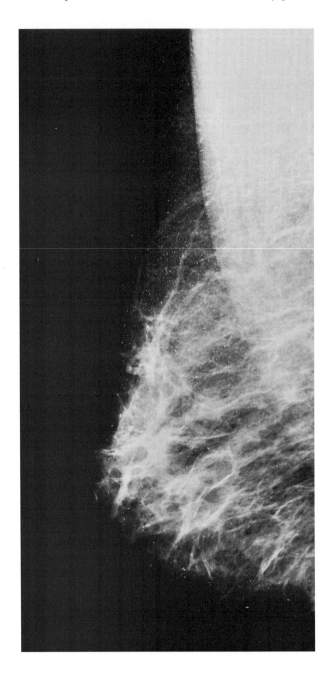

SOLUTION 4

If the artifacts are the result of dirt on the screen, the dirt should be visible on the screen when it is viewed on edge and under a strong light. The artifacts are more likely to be processing artifacts. Processing chemicals may contain small particles of precipitate that adhere to the film emulsion. The artifacts could also be caused by foreign particles in an automatic loading system (daylight loader) being deposited on the film by the vacuum handling system before development. These particles represent fine particulate material from deteriorating seals in the daylight loading equipment. When the particles are transported into the developer, they interfere with complete development of the film, causing fine "pick-off" artifacts.

QUESTIONS

1. Your facility has negotiated a service contract with a new processor chemical supply company. When the new chemistry is installed, the speed point on the sensitometric strip is 1.35 instead of 1.2 optical density. What should be done? Is the chemistry satisfactory?

2. A mobile van's on-board desktop processor was set to match the tank type processor at the breast center it services so that if the on-board processor fails, batch processing can occur. However, the speed of the mobile processor decreases during the week until it is usually 0.2 optical density lower on Friday than it was Monday. What could cause this?

3. A facility has found that their mean glandular dose is 215 mrad, above the 200 mrad allowed in that state.

They do not want to change screen/film combinations and cassettes because of the expense. The processor already has been modified to process film for 3 minutes. The film optical density of the ACR mammography accreditation phantom is 1.4 optimal density. What can be done to reduce the dose by about 8%?

4. What is the cause of small black dots on all the mammography films? The films developed just after the chemistry is changed do not have this artifact. This processor is used for emergency radiology as well as mammography.

5. A radiology center that performs very few mammograms has a tank-type processor. After the processor has been cleaned, contrast is poor, even though the speed set point on the sensitometric strip is within 0.10 optical density of the target value. What has caused the poor contrast?

ANSWERS

1. The chemistry is now more active than it was. If the base + fog is also higher, particularly if it is over 0.2 optical density, more starter may be needed. If the base + fog value is within 0.03 of the former base + fog (and is still below 0.2), then you should be pleased that you can slightly reduce the exposure to your patients. The new sensitometric speed set point should be based on an average of five sensitometric values for that set point. You may wish to have your mammography unit's service engineer adjust the automatic exposure control on his or her next visit to your facility.

2. If the replenishment developer is carried on the van already mixed, the van's movement and higher interior temperatures could cause excessive oxidation in the developer. To avoid this fluctuation, we mix our developer daily for the mobile van processor.

3. A slight rise in developer temperature, from 95 to 97°F (35–36°C), will increase film speed without affecting base + fog or contrast. The processor service engineer can make this adjustment. Temperatures up to 98°F (36.7°C) may be used for mammography if the facility has a high patient volume and the replenishment rate is set for at least 50 ml per 14 × 17 inch film (1560 cm²).

4. Because the processor is never turned off, the wash water sits, warm and stagnant, all day and night between cleanings. In this environment, small pieces of algae form and flake off the sides of the water tank during processing and become embedded in the soft gelatin of the developed film. In addition, the developer oxidizes more rapidly in this environment. Dropping chlorine tablets into the wash tank as a prophylactic measure is not recommended because the tablets crumble, leaving white particles on the film. An inexpensive desktop processor that is used exclusively for mammography is recommended.

5. The chemical supplier may be using the old replenishment developer to refill the tank after it has been drained and cleaned. The old replenishment developer is less active than fresh developer because it was mixed 1 month ago, but as it does not contain starter it will still be more active than the developer that has been drained. By adding about half the starter usually required for fresh chemistry, the old replenishment developer can probably be matched in speed to the sensitometer speed point. However, base + fog may be elevated, and contrast will be lower. When the processor is cleaned, both the developer and developer replenishment tanks should receive the newly mixed chemicals.

10

RADIATION DOSE

Women often ask, "How much radiation will I receive during my mammogram?" Concern with radiation exposure has led some women to refuse mammography or to refuse the additional views that are essential to resolve abnormalities seen on the initial images. This chapter is designed to help the reader answer questions that patients ask about radiation risk from mammography. It also provides information that will assist a mammography practice in keeping radiation doses as low as possible while maintaining good image quality. Some material has been discussed previously but is summarized again for emphasis.

DOSE MEASUREMENTS

Early in the history of mammography, exposure to the surface of the breast closest to the x-ray tube was used to characterize the amount of radiation received by the breast. The high attenuation coefficient of the parenchyma and its resultant absorption of the low-energy x-rays were not generally considered to be important factors until the late 1970s, when a controversy arose over mammography dose. In 1976, John Bailar (Bailar J. Mammography: a contrary view. Ann Intern Med 1976;84:77–84) maintained that as many cancers would be induced as were found by mammography, a hypothesis later nullified by recent mammography techniques that produced higher cancer discovery rates and lower doses. It was largely in response to the criticisms of Bailar and others that sophisticated research to determine actual mammography dosage was undertaken, and methods to diminish the dose were developed.

One such effort to determine actual dosage was directed by G. R. Hammerstein, who made use of material developed by D. R. White. This material, BR12, simulated the electron density of breast tissue. Hammerstein and his group devised a method to measure average absorbed dose in the glandular, at-risk portion of the breast, and they established that the dose varied with breast thickness, ratio of glandular to adipose tissue, and the radiation energy spectrum produced by the mammography unit. The tables and formulas derived from these experiments are used today to calculate the mean glandular dose (MGD). All breasts are assumed to have a 5-mm-thick envelope of skin and fat that surround the glandular tissue (Fig. 10.1). Because the glandular tissue is mixed with adipose tissue, breasts are characterized by the proportion of fat they contain relative to the amount of remaining glandular tissue. The attenuation coefficients for the various mixtures of breast tissue are then calculated and averaged. For example, a 4-cm thick 50% glandular breast that received 1 R[a] skin exposure at 26 kVp from a Mo anode mammography unit with a half value layer (HVL) of 0.3 mm Al would receive a MGD of 0.16 rad. Table 10.1 gives the multiplying factors that can be used to calculate dose from any skin exposure as long as breast compression is firm and the breast thickness, kVp, and HVL are known. Predominantly fatty breasts require conversion factors that are about 15% higher.

Clinical dose measurements can be made by the sharing of information between the technologist and medical physicist. The physicist can provide mR/mAs and half value layer measurements at the clinically relevant kVp,

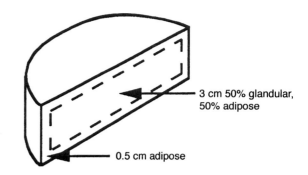

3 cm 50% glandular, 50% adipose

0.5 cm adipose

Figure 10.1. In Hammerstein's experiments, a hemicylinder of BR12 simulates a breast for which MGD was calculated.

---

[a]Roentgen (R) is the unit commonly used for exposure to radiation just as rad is used for absorbed dose. Scientific usage employs an international system of units (SI), coulombs/kg, and mGray: 1 R = 2.58 10^{-4} coulombs/kg, whereas 1 rad = 10 mGy. Because SI units are used almost exclusively in technical reports and common usage units are more familiar in clinical practice, we will use R and rad throughout this text.

Table 10.1.
Conversion of Skin Exposure to Mean Glandular Breast Dose
for Tissue That Is 50% Fatty and 50% Glandular

Anode/Filter	kVp	HVL	Breast Thickness					
			3 cm	4 cm	5 cm	6 cm	7 cm	8 cm
Mo/Mo[a]	25	0.3	0.21	0.16	0.13	0.10	0.09	
		0.32	0.22	0.17	0.13	0.11	0.09	
		0.34	0.23	0.18	0.14	0.12	0.10	
	26	0.3	0.21	0.16	0.13	0.10	0.09	
		0.32	0.22	0.17	0.13	0.11	0.09	
		0.34	0.22	0.17	0.14	0.12	0.10	
	27	0.32	0.22	0.17	0.14	0.11	0.10	
		0.34	0.23	0.18	0.14	0.12	0.10	
		0.36	0.25	0.19	0.15	0.13	0.11	
Mo/Rh[b]	26	0.34	0.24	0.18	0.15	0.12	0.10	
		0.36	0.25	0.19	0.16	0.13	0.11	
		0.38	0.26	0.20	0.16	0.14	0.12	
	27	0.36	0.25	0.20	0.16	0.13	0.11	
		0.38	0.26	0.20	0.17	0.14	0.12	
		0.40	0.27	0.21	0.17	0.14	0.12	
	28	0.38	0.26	0.20	0.17	0.14	0.12	
		0.40	0.27	0.21	0.17	0.14	0.12	
		0.42	0.28	0.22	0.18	0.15	0.13	
Rh/Rh[b]	26	0.36	0.25	0.20	0.16	0.14	0.12	
		0.38	0.27	0.21	0.17	0.14	0.12	
		0.40	0.28	0.22	0.18	0.15	0.13	
	27	0.38	0.27	0.21	0.17	0.15	0.12	
		0.40	0.28	0.22	0.18	0.15	0.13	
		0.42	0.29	0.23	0.19	0.16	0.14	
	28	0.38	0.27	0.21	0.18	0.15	0.13	
		0.40	0.28	0.22	0.18	0.15	0.13	
		0.42	0.29	0.23	0.19	0.16	0.14	
W/Rh[c]	25	0.43		0.23		0.16		0.12
		0.46		0.24		0.17		0.12
	27	0.46		0.24		0.17		0.12
		0.48		0.26		0.18		0.13
	29	0.47		0.25		0.17		0.13
		0.50		0.26		0.18		0.14
	31	0.48		0.26		0.18		0.14
		0.51		0.27		0.19		0.14
W/Ag[d]	33	0.6	0.39	0.32	0.27	0.23	0.20	
		0.62	0.40	0.32	0.27	0.23	0.20	
		0.64	0.41	0.33	0.28	0.24	0.21	
		0.66	0.41	0.34	0.29	0.24	0.21	

[a]From Wu X, Barnes GT, Tucker D. Spectral dependence of glandular tissue dose in screen/film mammography. Radiology 1991;179:143–148.
[b]From Wu X, Gingold EL, Barnes GT, Tucker DM. Normalized average glandular dose in molybdenum target-rhodium filter and rhodium target-rhodium filter mammography. Radiology 1994;193:83–89.
[c]Communication from Xizeng Wu, University of Alabama.
[d]Digital mammography systems only. From JM Tran, Trex Medical Systems.

allowing a table similar to Table 10.2 to be developed for each mammography unit at the facility.

Should the unit not have an Rh anode, the table will not require Rh/Rh entries. To calculate the MGD for a patient, the technologist must first record the mAs needed for each view, the kVp, anode, and filter used, and the thickness of the compressed breast. Armed with this information, and the half value layer supplied by the physicist, it is easy to use Table 10.1 to find the conversion factor for each view. For example, to calculate MGD, multiply the mAs by the mR/mAs entry in your physicist's Table 10.2 that matches the technique used. The product is the skin exposure in roentgens. Now find the HVL from Table 10.2 for the technique and anode/filter combination you used. In Table 10.1, find the correct anode/filter entry, kVp, and HVL for the exposure. The MGD conversion factor is multiplied by the skin exposure to obtain MGD. Note that in Table 10.1 the W/Rh and Rh/Rh data go to 31 and 28 kVp, respectively. Table 10.1 also includes data for a W target and silver (Ag) filter at high kVp; both techniques are used for digital but not screen/film mammography (see Chapter 13).

ACCURACY OF MEASUREMENTS

Because the estimated percentages of glandular and adipose tissue in a breast are purely subjective, as is the firmness of breast compression, calculation of MGD is an approximation. Should the technologist fail to record the kVp of the exposure, use of an approximate HVL will not produce a large error in the calculated dose. But should the breast thickness be under- or overestimated by 1 cm or more, the error in dose measurement will be significant.

Often a mathematical method engenders a mystique regarding its accuracy that is unrealistic. It is, therefore, inappropriate to make painstaking and time-consuming

Table 10.2.
Sample Physicist Data Needed to Calculate Mean Glandular Dose

Anode/Filter	kVp	HVL	mR/mAs
Mo/Mo	25	0.29	7.8
	26	0.31	8.3
	27	0.32	9.4
Mo/Rh	26	0.35	5.6
	27	0.37	6.8
	28	0.40	8.3
Rh/Rh	26	0.38	4.3
	27	0.40	5.2
	28	0.42	6.7

interpolation between HVL entries in Table 10.1, because it is only a guide to dose and not an absolute standard. Were state requirements to specify 200 mrad to a 4.5-cm breast phantom as the maximum MGD allowable per exposure, a measurement of 210 mrad would necessitate dose reduction but not decertification. A unit that produces more than 300 mrad/exposure to a 4.5-cm breast phantom is not performing quality mammography, however, and should not be certified.

One additional factor not covered by Table 10.1 or by most regulations is the optical density of the film produced by the exposure. A 20% increase in exposure produces less than a 0.2 optical density difference for most screen/film/processor combinations. If films are usually read at optical densities above 1.4, reducing the exposure by 20% will cause the film optical density to decrease to a level that still remains above 1.2, a level that is still acceptable. If the MGD to a phantom is found to be 210 mrad, the optical density of the film may be lowered to lower the dose, provided the optical density at the chest wall remains above 1.2.

MAMMOGRAPHY CARCINOGENESIS

Regulations on mammography dosage are based on the doses at an "average" facility when imaging a standard phantom. Limits are set by the equipment and not by the possible biological effects of ionizing radiation. This "average" dose has been used in studies of radiation exposure to calculate the excess numbers of breast cancers that might result from exposure to a large population. Among the populations investigated were Japanese women who were exposed to high-energy radiation during the atomic bombing of Hiroshima and Nagasaki, women who had pulmonary tuberculosis and were exposed to the radiation of multiple fluoroscopic examinations, and women who had postpartum mastitis treated with radiation. These studies and others helped to predict the number of excess cancers that might be expected from mammography. The risk of radiation-induced carcinogenesis varies with age. Although the calculations assume no differences between high- and low-energy radiation, between large and small doses, or between short and long intervals of multiple exposures, it is known that radiation-induced damage varies widely according to these factors; ignoring them leads to overestimation of carcinogenic risk of mammography.

Epidemiologists have established that mammograms begun after age 50 contribute to 4/100,000 excess deaths from breast cancer by age 75. The benefit-to-risk ratio increases with advancing age because the breasts of women

50 years or older are less sensitive to radiation than those of younger women and because the risk of naturally occurring breast cancer increases with increasing age.

Benefit-to-risk ratio is calculated by comparing the number of women saved from death because a cancer was detected in their mammograms with the number of women who may have developed a radiation-induced breast cancer and subsequently have died from it. Because breast cancers detected at an early stage have a high cure rate, the benefit-to-risk ratio is highest for women older than 50, in whom the incidence of breast cancer is greatest and whose breast tissue contains more adipose than glandular tissue, which eases early detection. The American College of Radiology, American Cancer Society, and National Cancer Institute recommend annual or biennial screening mammograms between ages 40 and 50, with annual screening mammograms thereafter. Although screening mammography is usually not recommended before age 40, a woman under 40 whose mother died of bilateral premenopausal breast cancer or who has had a personal history of breast cancer should consult her physician about the benefits of screening mammography.

MAMMOGRAPHY EQUIPMENT: EFFECT ON DOSE

Dose is affected by many components of mammography equipment. Their particular contributions to dose will now be discussed, along with methods to limit the dose (Fig. 10.2).

The generator of the mammography unit affects the energy spectrum and the output, both of which affect dose. The energy spectrum depends, in part, on the type of electrical power supplied to the x-ray tube. A single-phase, rectified voltage pulse will generate more low-energy radiation than a single-phase, high-frequency voltage pulse. The lower energy photons are more likely to be absorbed by the breast, increasing the absorbed dose. Furthermore, a low output of x-rays will cause the duration of exposure to be prolonged. The resultant failure of the film reciprocity law will necessitate a higher dose than that required for a shorter exposure to achieve equal film darkening. To keep the dose to a minimum, single-phase voltage with a high-frequency generator or three-phase voltage with either a six-pulse or high-frequency generator is preferred.

Anode materials have already been discussed in relation to their effect on contrast. Some mammography manufacturers have combined W or Rh anodes with Rh filters to increase breast penetration and to reduce dose. Increasing the filtration of a Mo anode tube increases the HVL and reduces dose (as long as sufficient output remains to avoid film reciprocity law failure) but also reduces contrast.

The size of the focal spot also affects dose because of film reciprocity law failure. If the focal spot is conceived as a hose through which the electrons heading toward the anode must squeeze, it becomes apparent why a smaller focal spot causes a longer exposure than a larger focal spot.

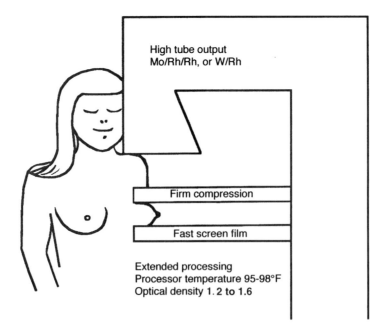

Figure 10.2. Factors that contribute to decreased patient dose.

The radiation dose required to expose different screen/film combinations may vary by as much as 100%. The same is true of development time and temperature. Not every facility can make use of processor dose-saving strategies, but appropriate selection of screens and film can be achieved in any facility. When undertaking the clinical testing of fast, lower dose screen/film combinations, it must be determined whether the increased mottle in glandular portions of the breast interferes with the resolution of small structures. It is essential to look for possible degradation of images by comparing serial studies of the same breast imaged with the new and old screen/film combinations.

Compression should not be overlooked as a dose-saving strategy. Patients may be more accepting of firm compression when they are made to understand that a decrease in breast thickness of only 0.5 cm can reduce the dose to their breasts significantly. If the skin exposure for a 4.5-cm thick breast is 1.43 R, it falls to 1.07 R when the breast is compressed to a thickness of 4 cm. When converted to MGD with multiplying factors of 0.15 and 0.17, respectively, the 4.5-cm thick breast receives 215 mrad, whereas the 4-cm-thick breast receives 182 mrad, a savings of 15%.

The film cassette also contributes to dose. Manufacturers continually change the design and composition of their cassettes. When accepting delivery of new cassettes, compare them with those that are to be replaced. Identical manual exposures of a phantom should not produce significantly different optical densities for the old and new cassettes. The manufacturer should be notified if a new cassette produces a film whose optical density is 0.15 less than the film produced by the old cassette. Of course, the screen uniformity test and screen/film contact test should be performed on all new screens before they are accepted.

OTHER DOSE CONSIDERATIONS

Many decisions made in radiological practice affect the lifetime radiation dose received by a patient. Because patients who undergo screening generally return to the same facility for yearly examinations, consistent, albeit small, dose savings can multiply into large ones over the lifetime of the patient. Although yearly screening mammography of women younger than 40 must be treated on an individualized basis, a personal history of breast cancer is a reason for the immediate initiation of yearly screening without regard to age.

As will be discussed in Chapter 11, a critical review of discarded films may lead to a decrease in the number that must be repeated. When mammography is under-

taken on a new patient or on one whose previous radiographs are unavailable, ideally, one exposure of one breast should be made, processed, and evaluated technically before any additional exposures are made. If the patient's breast is found to be predominantly fatty or predominantly dense, adjustments in the automatic exposure control or the anode/filter combination can be made at the expense of only one excess exposure. Radiological evaluation of the standard views may lead to extra views for additional evaluation of a questionable area. A patient who objects to additional views may consent to them when she is shown her initial mammograms, and the technologist explains to her what will be achieved. This should not increase anxiety if the technologist uses an easily understood phrase like, "this area is not spread out enough, so we are going to change your position to see the area more clearly." By making the patient a partner in the examination rather than an object, the technologist may gain more cooperation and achieve a better diagnostic study.

Every facility should invest in 24 × 30 cm grids and cassettes for imaging large breasts, rather than performing multiple exposures using 18 × 24 cm cassettes. Not only does the added number of radiographs complicate the evaluation, but many parts of the breast receive two and sometimes three times the absorbed dose required for a single radiograph of the entire breast. About 10% of our patients require large cassettes.

Quality control testing results in lower doses by eliminating the causes of repeat films: excessive dose, caused by output or kVp that is too low or films that are too dark, and suboptimal film processing.

MAGNIFICATION AND DOSE

As we have emphasized, the magnification view should always be performed as a noncontact compression spot view, not only to reduce dose but also to reduce scatter and optimize compression. In a recent article (see Liu et al. under "Suggested Readings"), the MGD from a magnified view was calculated to be 7–25% lower than that from a nonmagnified view because the entire breast was not irradiated and because the shorter distance between the x-ray tube and skin caused attenuation in the breast to change more rapidly for the magnified view than it did at the longer source-to-object distance used for the nonmagnified view. Table 10.3 provides MGD conversion tables for Mo/Mo magnified views. An unmagnified contact spot view of an area of interest also reduces the dose to the rest of the breast.

Table 10.3.
Mean Glandular Dose Conversions for Magnified,
Coned-Down Mo/Mo, Gridless Exposures

	HVL	\multicolumn{5}{c}{Breast Thickness}
		3 cm	4 cm	5 cm	6 cm	7 cm
26 kVp	0.30	0.19	0.14	0.11	0.09	0.07
	0.32	0.20	0.15	0.12	0.09	0.08
	0.34	0.21	0.16	0.12	0.10	0.08
28 kVp	0.32	0.21	0.15	0.12	0.09	0.08
	0.34	0.22	0.16	0.13	0.10	0.08
	0.36	0.23	0.17	0.13	0.10	0.09

Extracted from Reference 2 for 50/50 breast.

Suggested Readings

Feig SA, Hendrick RE. Risk, benefit, and controversies in mammography screening. In: Haus AG, Yaffe MJ, eds. Syllabus: a categorical course in physics. Technical aspects of breast imaging, 3rd ed. Radiological Society of North America 80th Annual Meeting, Nov 27–Dec 2, 1994.

This very detailed review describes the different statistical risk models for radiation-induced cancer at different ages. It also reviews the benefits from screening based on clinical trials, including those in Sweden, Holland, Italy, United Kingdom, and Canada.

Liu R, Goodsitt M, Chan H-P. Normalized average glandular dose in magnification mammography. Radiology 1995;199:27–32.

This article discusses why magnification mammography yields less dose than nonmagnified mammography. It also provides tables for calculating MGD that are more comprehensive than Table 10.3.

Moskowitz MM. Benefits and risks. In: Bassett LW, Gold RH, eds. Breast cancer detection: mammography and other methods in breast imaging, 2nd ed. New York: Grune & Stratton, 1987.

Everything you ever wanted to know about how mammography benefit and risk are calculated. This excellent article includes a glossary of terms and a complete reference list.

PROBLEM 1

This dense 6-cm thick breast (*left*) was imaged with an old 3 phase unit (Mo/Mo) that was underpowered. To increase penetration, the kVp was 28 with a HVL of 0.36 mm Al. The exposure required was 2.4 R. Because the image was underpenetrated, the patient was moved to a new high-frequency unit and reimaged (*right*), using Mo/Mo, at 26 kVp, HVL = 0.32 with an exposure of 2.8 R. Did the MGD increase for the second exposure? Is this an acceptable dose according to Mammography Quality Standards Act?

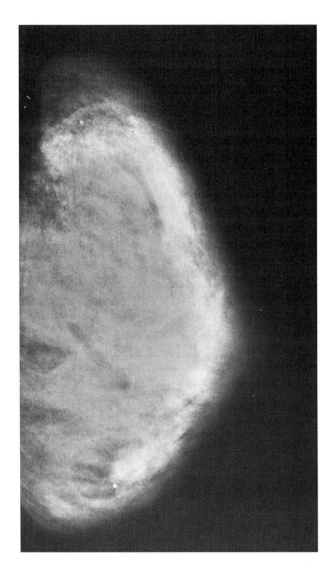
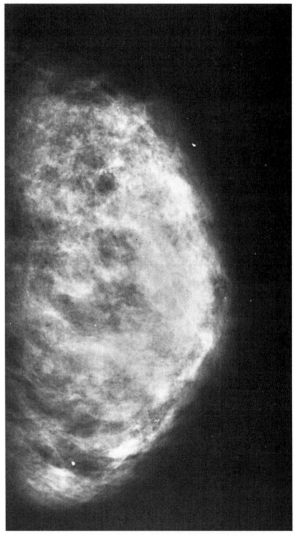

SOLUTION 1

In Table 10.1, there is no entry for 28 kVp. However, each kVp increases the MGD factor by 0.01 so that for 28 kVp, HVL = 0.36, and for a 6-cm thick breast, the conversion factor is 0.14. This gives a MGD of 336 mrad. For the second unit, the conversion factor is 0.11, giving a MGD of 308 mrad despite the higher exposure. The same low kVp technique on the old machine would have required an even higher exposure because the tube output would have been less and the film reciprocity law failure would have increased the exposure needed for the same film darkening.

Although the Mammography Quality Standards Act does not require that all MGD values be below 300 mrad, it does require that the dose needed to expose an American College of Radiography mammography accreditation phantom to an optical density between 1.2 and 1.6 be below 300 mrad. Because the phantom is 4.5 cm thick, the two units could probably expose the phantom, using the techniques provided in the problem, to 0.6 and 0.7 R, respectively. Because the multiplying factors for a 4-cm-thick breast exposed with these two techniques are 0.20 and 0.17, respectively, the doses for the phantom would be 120 mrad and 119 mrad, respectively—well below the 300 mrad limit.

PROBLEM 2

A woman with predominantly fatty 4-cm-thick breasts is imaged at 25 kVp and 65 mAs. Unfortunately, the technologist left the automatic exposure control sensor in the third position, so the exposure was terminated too soon, resulting in a mammogram (*left*) with an optical density of only 1.0 at the chest wall. A second exposure was made with the automatic exposure control correctly positioned, resulting in an optical density of 1.4 at the chest wall (*right*). The technique was 25 kVp and 90 mAs. The medical physicist provided the following table for the mammography unit (similar to Table 10.2).

	kVp	HVL	mR/mAs
Mo/Mo	25	0.30	9.0
	26	0.31	10.0
	27	0.33	10.8
Rh/Rh	26	0.37	6.0
	27	0.39	7.0
	28	0.41	8.5

Calculate the increase in dose required by the darker film.

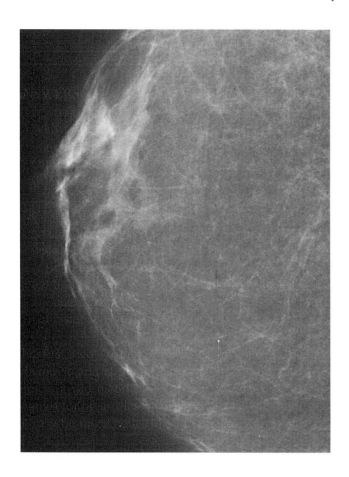
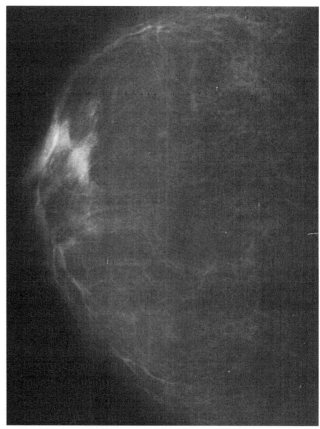

SOLUTION 2

Just as in Solution 1 there was a failure to convert the MGD in Table 10.1 to a value more representative of a dense breast (about 25% decrease in the MGD factor) so will this solution fail to consider the effect of a fatty breast on the MGD factor (a 12% increase). Because we are comparing two doses for the same breast rather than calculating an absolute dose, this short cut is acceptable. Therefore, from Table 10.2, using the 25 kVp entry, the skin exposure at 65 mAs is 585 mR, whereas at 90 mAs it is 810 mR. Because the MGD conversion factor is 0.16 for both exposures, the difference in dose is 94 mrad vs. 130 mrad, a 40% increase in dose to obtain the correct optical density.

PROBLEM 3

A 65-year-old patient has never had a mammogram. She is surprised that the technologist pulls her breast and then compresses it and protests the discomfort and indignity. As a result, the technologist, who is relatively inexperienced, is inhibited from applying full compression. The following exposures were made on a Mo/Mo unit at 26 kVp.

	mAs	Thickness (cm)
LCC	228	6.0
RCC	207	6.0
LMLO	395	7.0
RMLO	305	6.5

Using the physicist tables from Problem 2, what dose did each breast receive? What dose would have been received had the breast been compressed 1 cm more for all views? What dose would each have received if it had been compressed 1 cm more (i.e., the LCC compressed to 5 cm thickness) and imaged with Rh/Rh? (Assume mAs values are 30% less for Rh/Rh.)

SOLUTION 3

Let us create a table to help compare these values.

	cm	mR	MGD Factor	MGD (mrad)
Mo/Mo, LCC	6.0	2280	0.11	251
RCC	6.0	2070	0.11	228
LMLO	7.0	3950	0.09	356
RMLO	6.5	3050	0.10	305

Therefore, the right breast received a total of 513 mrad, and the left breast received 607 mrad.

If the breast could have been compressed 1 cm more on all views, the mAs needed would have been reduced by 50%. The table then would look like this:

	cm	mR	MGD Factor	MGD (mrad)
Mo/Mo, LCC	5.0	1140	0.13	148
RCC	5.0	1035	0.13	135
LMLO	6.0	1975	0.11	217
RMLO	5.5	1525	0.12	183

Now the right breast receives a total of 318 mrad and the left 365 mrad.

If Rh/Rh is used, the table now looks like this:

	cm	mAs[a]	mR	MGD Factor	MGD (mrad)
LCC	5.0	79.8	479	0.17	81
RCC	50.0	72.5	435	0.17	74
LMLO	6.0	138.3	830	0.14	116
RMLO	5.5	106.8	640	0.15	96

[a]mAs reduced by 50% because of greater compression and 30% because of the Rh/Rh combination. Total is 35%.

Therefore, the right breast receives a total of 170 mrad, and the left breast receives 197 mrad, a factor of 3 compared with the dose received by the breasts when they were not fully compressed and were imaged with Mo/Mo.

PROBLEM 4

Calcifications near a suspicious area of increased density were imaged with two standard contact views (**A** and **B**) and two magnification views (**C** and **D**). The techniques are given below.

	kVp (HVL = 0.3)	mAs	Breast Thickness (cm)
Contact views (Mo/Mo)			
Craniocaudal	25	48	4
Oblique	25	96	5
	kVp (HVL = 0.34)		
Magnified views			
Craniocaudal	28	25	3
Lateral	28	48	4

Tube output at 25 kVp is 10 mR/mAs for the large focal spot. For the small focal spot, the output measured at the skin for a magnified view is 15 mR/mAs. What is the total MGD to the suspicious area?

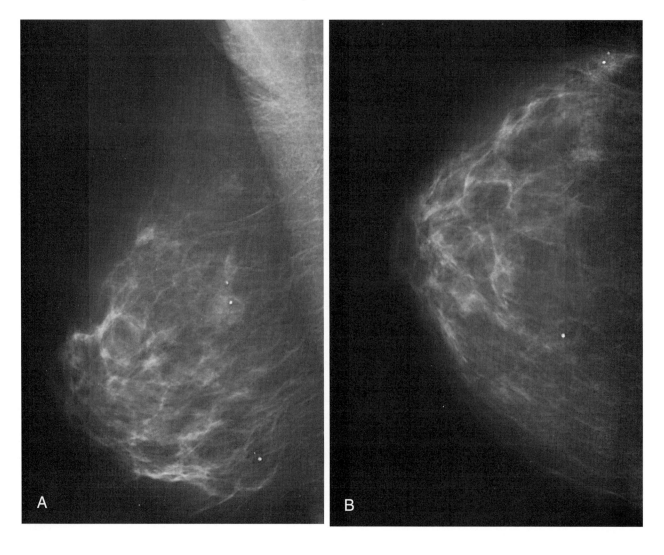

PROBLEM 4—Continued

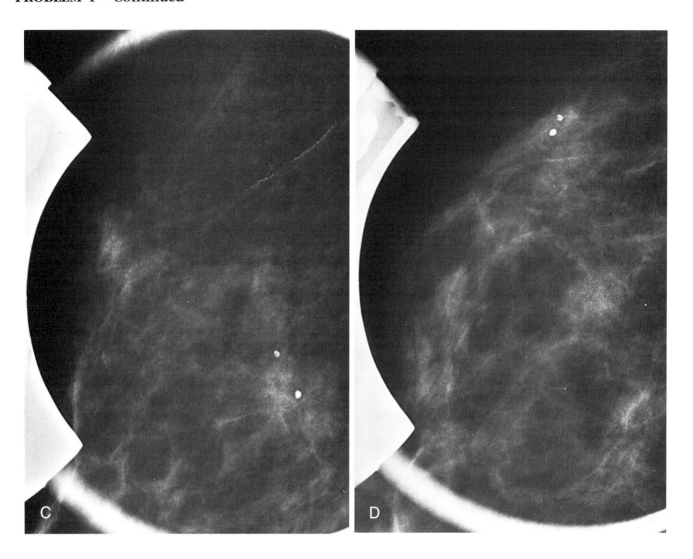

SOLUTION 4

	Multiplying Factor	Exposure (mR)	Dose (mrad)
Contact views			
Craniocaudal	0.16	480	77
Oblique	0.13	960	125
Magnification views (see Table 10.3)			
Cranicaudal	0.22	375	83
Lateral	0.16	720	115.4

The total dose is 400 mrad. This is acceptable because of the benefit that diagnosis of an early stage, clinically occult cancer can contribute to the life expectancy of the patient.

QUESTIONS

1. Rank these dose reduction methods according to their effect on mammography quality: faster screen/film combination, Rh/Rh or W/Rh, increased kVp, greater compression, extended processing, greater x-ray output, lighter films, higher processing temperature.

2. A mammogram from a 35-year-old patient with a family history of breast cancer showed a mass that was solid on ultrasound examination. Because it is classified as BI RADS diagnosis 5, biopsy is recommended. Should she have a stereotactically guided core biopsy, requiring seven to nine x-ray exposures?

3. A 50-year-old woman with very large breasts would require two 24 × 30 cm films for each view, or each breast could be imaged with four 18 × 24 cm films. Because each view is similar to a spot compression view, each breast would be compressed to a lesser thickness than if it had been compressed in its entirety in a single view. For dose savings, which size film should be used?

4. A 30-year-old man with a lump behind his nipple has been sent to your facility for mammography. Because of his age, should he receive an ultrasound examination instead?

5. A patient with silicone implants has mammograms. Compared with a woman without implants, what dose to each breast can be expected?

ANSWERS

1. With respect to image quality, in order of diminishing quality:
   (a) greater compression (if possible)
   (b) extended processing
   (c) greater x-ray output (i.e., a different mammography unit)
   (d) higher processing temperature (up to 98°F)
   (e) Rh/Rh or W/Rh (at 26 kVp)
   (f) increased kVp (up to 27 kVp)
   (g) lighter films (down to 1.2 optical density at the chest wall)
   (h) faster screen/film combination

The first two (a and b) will improve image quality, whereas c and d should have no effect on quality (except to avoid motion for c). Both e and f will degrade contrast for breasts less than 5.5 cm thick. Quantum mottle may be more noticeable for choices g and h.

2. She can avoid the x-ray exposures by having an ultrasonically guided core biopsy. However, because the x-ray core biopsy is diagnostic, x-ray exposures are not as great a concern as they would be in a screening examination, which is repeated yearly.

3. Because of the x-ray exposure to overlapping tissue when four films are required, two 24 × 30 cm films are recommended. Compressing one-fourth of the breast while the other three-fourths is below the breast support platform is difficult.

4. Because men are not screened for breast cancer, diagnostic mammography at any age is recommended. Although an ultrasound examination may aid diagnosis, it is rarely used alone except for women younger than 30 with very dense breasts.

5. Because both an Eklund (pinch or implant displacement) technique and a manual exposure of the silicone implant are obtained for each view, the patient receives two times the dose that was received by a woman without silicone implants.

11

QUALITY CONTROL

The reader who is aware of the quality control procedures mandated by Mammography Quality Standards Act (MQSA) may feel overwhelmed by their complexity and the time they require. Even one who is knowledgeable about the procedures may not have experienced an MQSA inspection and may be unprepared for the attention to detail that is demanded. This chapter offers suggestions concerning how quality control can be performed most efficiently within MQSA guidelines and describes how to avoid the pitfalls that could arise during an inspection.

TECHNOLOGIST'S QUALITY ASSURANCE

The radiologic technologist should obtain quality assurance (QA) record forms from the film supplier. These will provide a format for QA record keeping. Some procedures that are performed daily or weekly require a check-off form. QA record forms located in the darkroom and at the view box will remind personnel about the need to clean the darkroom daily and the view box weekly. In the event that an autoloader is used, the darkroom must still be cleaned no less than biweekly because it continues to be used to load the film into canisters and to expose the sensitometric strips. At our facility, the radiologist is responsible for cleaning the view box and for recording this activity on the appropriate check-off form. A third QA form for screen cleaning should list all cassettes by their number and provide columns for weekly check-off.

Although processor QC is the most onerous procedure required, it is the one that most affects mammography quality. The QC technologist should arrive 30 minutes before the first patient, replace the crossover rollers, and start the processor. Because it must be ensured that the patient's prior radiographs are available and that the mammography rooms are unlocked and ready, the technologist will be occupied until the correct processing temperature is reached. The QC technologist should set aside 15 minutes to expose a sensitometric strip, process it, and evaluate the results. Although automatic strip readers are now available, their use should not preclude the technologist's assurance that the processor is operating within 0.15 optical density of the established average value. When these limits are exceeded, the technologist must record what corrective action was taken before processing the films of patients.

Monthly phantom images also require annotating corrective actions if background density or exposure are outside recommended limits (Fig. 11.1). Some MQSA inspectors recommend exposing a second phantom image after correcting the problem that caused the out-of-limits outcome.

We have found that the monthly tests require less time to accomplish when they are performed on the same day rather than piecemeal in the intervals between patient examinations. Because of the high volume at our facility, we perform the retake analysis monthly. Therefore, 30 minutes per mammography unit is set aside monthly to image the phantom, complete the appropriate checklist, and perform retake analysis. Data recording the number of films used per month, required for retake analysis, are automatically recorded by some autoloader systems or can be estimated from the number of boxes of film consumed during the month.

Fixer retention, performed quarterly, can be made to coincide with the quarterly review of the QA records by the radiologist, which may help remind the technologist that it is time for the quarterly QA review. Minutes of these reviews should be kept and initialed by the radiologist in charge of the breast center.

Semiannual tests (darkroom fog, film-screen contact, and compression pressure monitoring) require 1 hour per mammography unit. The analysis of the film-screen contact images should not be hurried. If possible, screen cleaning, which should be performed weekly, should directly precede this test. The results can be recorded on the screen cleaning form that lists the numbers of the screens and cassettes. The first time this test is performed, a manual technique that provides a mesh optical density over 0.7 is needed (Fig. 11.2). If the sensitometer shows that changes in optical density occur with small changes in position, a larger aperture (the black button with a

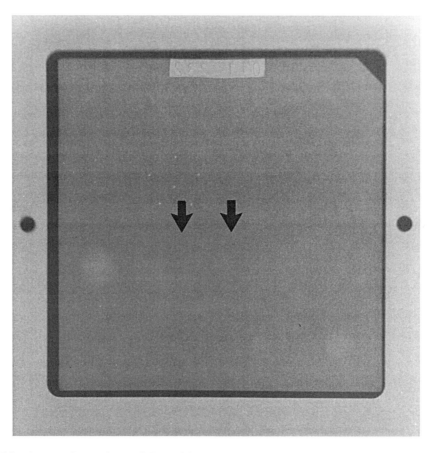

Figure 11.1. This phantom image is too light and has processor roller marks (*arrows*) running parallel to rollers.

hole through which light passes) will be needed. Some contact meshes have radiopaque dots in the center. If your mesh has such a dot, the optical density behind it should be at least 2.5. It will save time if you record the manual technique for both large and small cassettes (exposure may differ), the kVp, and the mammography unit used. We do not use the 2-cm clear plastic slab in addition to the mesh when testing screen/film contact.

We estimate that the minimum time needed by the technologist for QA per year is equivalent to approximately 19 8-hour days. For a facility with four mammography units, this increases to 27 days. Other record keeping, if performed by the technologist instead of the facility manager, can increase this estimate by 50%.

PHYSICIST'S QUALITY ASSURANCE

When MQSA was first implemented, physicists estimated that complete surveys would require 1–3 days per mammography unit. Most physicists now require less than 1 day to complete an inspection. Physicists using computer programs to prompt them during the survey generally require more time at the facility but less time for writing a final report compared with physicists who transcribe their results and enter them into a computer program off-

line. In the latter case, a complete survey, excluding off-premises analysis of results, can be performed in less than 4 hours if the mammography technologist can assist by processing films.

The physicist may wish to begin by inspecting the technologist's QA reports because they may reveal equipment problems that need special attention. The physicist should be particularly careful to check that all processor and phantom image results that are beyond accepted limits are documented with an explanation of the action taken. The technique that was used for the technologist's QA phantom images may be duplicated for the physicist's phantom images so long as background optical density is between 1.2 and 1.6. The technologist's QA evaluation of the mammographic unit assembly should have an itemized list of each item tested, and the physicist's unit assembly evaluation should have the same. The physicist who is also previewing the MQSA inspection should confirm that the MQSA permit is displayed in the patient waiting room and that documentation concerning training and continuing medical education credits for the radiologist, technologist, and physicist are available. This review of MQSA documents may take up to 1 hour, particularly at a new facility.

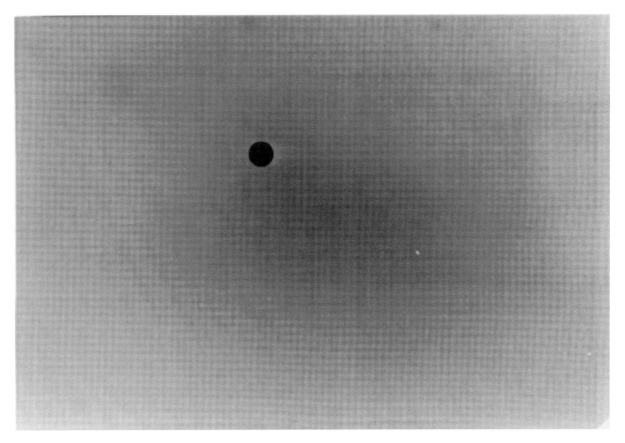

Figure 11.2. Screen/film contact test shows a large dark area below and to the right of the center black dot. If optical density were darker, this deficit in screen/film contact would be much more obvious (see "Problem 2").

During the equipment survey, the physicist should try to group similar tests together so that test equipment needed for several tests can be used at one time rather than intermittently. In addition to the tests required by the MQSA, we measure mR/mAs and output linearity, which enable us to provide a look-up table so that patient doses can be estimated from the recorded mAs, kVp, and breast thickness (see Chapter 10). Because narrow beam geometry is used for these tests, it is efficient to measure half value layer immediately after the mR/mAs is tested. MQSA inspectors expect at least three measurements at different clinically relevant kVps, with zero filtration and additional measurements with three thicknesses of aluminum that include 0.3 and 0.4 mm at each kVp.

The physicist's tests of kVp should repeat the kVp values used to test half value layer. At least three measurements at one kVp must be included. If a Mo/Rh, Rh/Rh, or W/Rh unit is being surveyed, and the physicist's noninvasive kVp meter is not calibrated for these anode/filter combinations, the physicist should be certain to specify in the report that the generator voltage supplied to the Mo anode is the same voltage that was supplied to the W or Rh anodes.

Automatic exposure control (AEC) must be tested using three thicknesses of breast equivalent material (Lucite or BR12) at one clinical kVp already tested for half value layer and kVp. The 4-cm-thick slab should then be reimaged at the other two kVps. The large (24 × 30 cm) cassettes and grid should also be tested in the same way, and all anode/filter combinations tested. The report should include mAs, kVp, thickness, and optical density. Magnification tests need not be as extensive but should include 2- and 4-cm breast thicknesses at the highest kVp tested. For magnification tests, the grid should be excluded. The amount of variation in mAs should be reported for density settings of +1 and −1. Three exposures at the same density setting, kVp, and breast thickness should be made. For these last two tests, mAs can be reported rather than the optical density of the exposed film.

While the grid is absent, after the AEC magnification test, we measure breast compression and the other unit assembly data. If possible, we image the normally reciprocating grid while it is stationary, particularly during acceptance testing, to ensure that the grid septi are intact.

The collimation assessment can be done without reversing the top film. Coins placed at each chest wall corner, without the compression paddle in place, and a coin taped to the compression paddle should suffice for all three sides and the compression paddle alignment tests. These films can be processed at the same time as the AEC tests and the phantom image(s). If Mo/Rh or Rh/Rh, W/Rh are available, phantom images of these combinations should be made at the kVp that is in clinical use.

We perform our focal spot measurements by placing two line pair phantoms perpendicular to each other in the American College of Radiology mammography accreditation phantom with the pink insert removed. With the AEC at −2, a sufficiently light image results; both width and length resolution may be reported from one film. The small focal spot is measured without the grid in place but with similar geometry.

Screen uniformity is checked once a year. A manual technique, derived from a preliminary AEC exposure, must achieve a sufficiently dark optical density (1.4 is ideal) for testing (Fig. 11.3). The average optical density for each cassette is tabulated according to the cassette number. Before leaving the facility, the physicist should make sure that each screen's identification number is shown on each image. If it does not, correct the position of the number, reexpose the cassette, and check the image again.

The physicist may have a preference regarding whether to complete the entire analysis at the facility or to analyze the results off-site in a more contemplative atmosphere. If the entire analysis is completed on-site, the mammography room will not be available for patients while it is underway. This actually increases the cost of the physicist's survey because of the resultant absence of patient imaging services. However, if the physicist immediately interviews the radiologist at the conclusion of the survey and identifies or corrects out of range parameters, the additional cost will be justified by improved patient service.

Figure 11.3. Irregular structure in this image was present for each 18 × 24 cm cassette test. Either the grid or the breast support device is at fault.

MQSA INSPECTION

Most MQSA inspectors have been well trained to perform a limited subset of the physicist's tests and to rigorously check QA records and personnel qualifications. They are not trained to be amenable to compromises in MQSA regulations. They report infringements according to three levels of severity. A level 1 response would imply that the radiologist or technologist is poorly trained in mammography or that the equipment gives more than 300 mrad mean glandular dose. A facility that receives a level 1 citation will not be licensed to perform mammography. A level 2 response indicates that the facility has a problem with its processor or other equipment or with its record keeping. A facility receiving a level 2 citation must respond within 30 days with a letter describing how the problem has been corrected.

Most facilities receive level 3 warnings citing less severe problems that must be rectified by the next inspection. The following are the most common level 3 problems cited.

1. The mammogram report is not in the patient's film jacket. Facilities with computer generated reports must be able to show that reports can be obtained on demand.
2. There is no systematic way of tracing patient outcomes for patients recommended for biopsy.
3. Technologist, radiologist, or physicist continuing medical education credits are not documented by certificates.
4. Radiologist and technologist licenses are not displayed in a patient area.
5. When the results of QA tests are beyond normal limits, no explanation of the causes and solutions are given.
6. Cassette numbers do not show on the films when testing for screen/film contact.
7. Roller marks are present on phantom images.
8. Maximum compression values are not written on compression test tabulation.
9. kVps tested do not match the AEC and phantom imaging kVp determined by the physicist.
10. The physicist did not tabulate the cassette numbers and optical density values when testing for uniformity and artifacts.

11. Optical density of $+1$ and -1 was not tested during AEC evaluation.
12. AEC was not tested across different kVps.
13. The small focal spot was not tested.
14. The unit assembly evaluation was not itemized.
15. No quality control test summary was included with the physicist's report.
16. The number of mammograms read by the radiologist is not documented.

Before final MQSA requirements are issued, the tests may be simplified and the number and required documentation reduced. The spirit of compliance may improve when rules are made more flexible and when radiologists receive more encouragement to self-monitor their practices.

Suggested Readings

Farria DM, Bassett LW, Kimme-Smith C, DeBruhl N. Mammography quality assurance from A to Z. RadioGraphics 1994;14:371–385.

This short article summarizes the radiologic technologist's QA responsibilities, patient positioning, image labeling, and the responsibilities of the medical physicist. The qualifications of the radiologist and the required patient follow-up and outcome assessment procedures are described.

Hendrick RE, Paquelet JR. Is the mammography quality standards act worth the cost? Radiology 1995;197:53A–57A, 1996;199:285–287 (response).

This article is critical of the MQSA inspection process. It will solace those who have had a negative experience at an MQSA inspection.

Mourad WG. Mammography quality standards act of 1992. Facility inspection procedures. Center for Devices of Radiological Health, Division of Mammography Quality and Radiation Programs, Sep 9, 1994 (draft).

This document will no doubt soon be succeeded by a new one; the reader may have to call Center for Devices of Radiological Health or the Food and Drug Administration to obtain it. It lists the questions asked by the MQSA inspector during a visit to a facility. It is invaluable as a checklist to determine if all MQSA requirements have been met.

PROBLEM 1

Is this an adequate phantom image? Critique it as you would a patient image (see "Problem 1" in Chapter 3).

SOLUTION 1

No. It illustrates poor processing, inept film handling, and dirty screens. The optical density is sufficient. Film scratches at the top of the film may be the result of sliding the film against a rough surface. In addition, either pick-off (from the processor) or screen dirt is present as small white dots over most of the image. At the bottom of the image, a light area obscuring the image of the smaller masses in the phantom probably results from uneven pressure near the edges of the rollers.

PROBLEM 2

Should the speck of dirt on the right side of the cassette be removed and the cassette used immediately for clinical imaging?

SOLUTION 2

The screen should be cleaned and the cassette reloaded with film and allowed to remain undisturbed for at least 15 minutes before retesting. The visualized small areas of poor screen/film contact usually result from air trapped between the screen and film that dissipate during these 15 minutes. If the mesh image is not significantly improved, the cassette should be replaced.

PROBLEM 3

This darkroom fog image was obtained. The part of the phantom covered during the test has an optical density of 1.5, whereas the right half of the phantom, which was uncovered during the test, has an optical density of 1.85. Is this a satisfactory test for darkroom fog or should it be repeated?

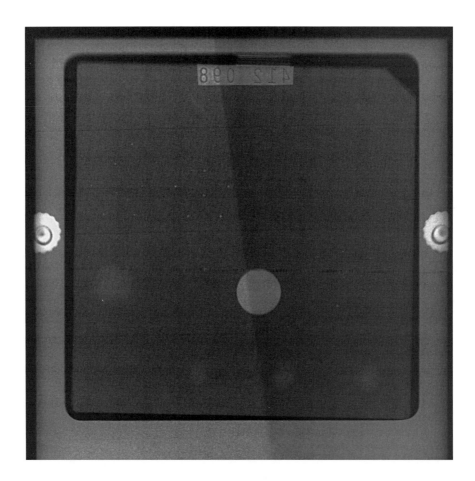

SOLUTION 3

The test was performed correctly, but darkroom fog was excessive. Either (*a*) the darkroom light is the wrong color, (*b*) the darkroom light is from a fluorescent tube behind a red glass filter and the red glass does not cover the fluorescent light, or (*c*) there are significant leaks around the door or the processor in the darkroom. Once the problem has been corrected, the darkroom fog test should be repeated.

PROBLEM 4

The screen uniformity test was performed on the 24 × 30 cm cassettes using a 2-cm piece of Lucite. All cassettes have this striped pattern and white dot (*arrow*). What could cause these artifacts? (Note this is a partial image of the 24 × 30 film; the bottom of the image is at the chest wall.)

SOLUTION 4

The stripes were originally thought to be grid related. However, on this mammography unit, the grid can be slid out of the way, leaving the cassette tunnel in place. Reimaging the Lucite slab, without the grid, the lines were still present. Therefore, they were due to the carbon fiber construction of the cassette tunnel. The white dot was a spatter of contrast material that had adhered to the Lucite slab when it was used for other calibration tests in the interventional fluoroscopy room.

PROBLEM 5

The two images below represent an x-ray/light field/compression paddle alignment test. **A.** Chest wall side of the 24 × 30 cassette resting on top of cassette tunnel, which held the film shown in **B**. *Solid arrows*, edge of compression paddle; *open arrows*, coin attached to edge of the compression paddle. Assuming that the side of the x-ray field farthest from the chest wall is properly aligned, does the alignment of this x-ray equipment meet minimum MQSA regulations?

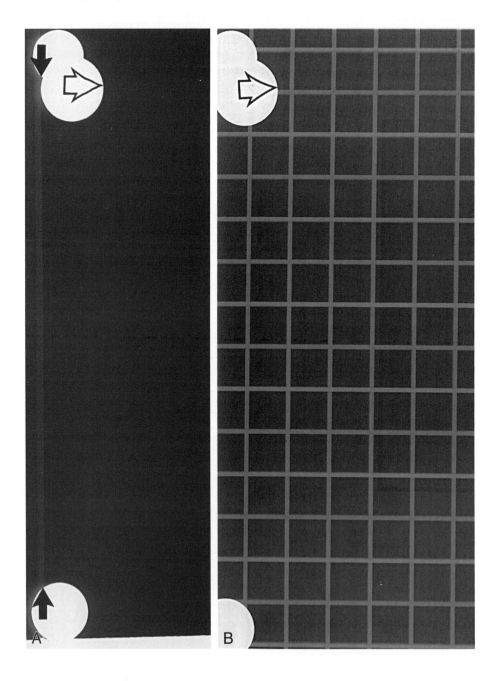

SOLUTION 5

Yes. The compression paddle is well aligned with the edge of the image receptor. The right to left deviation of the x-ray/light field is within 2% of the SID.

QUESTIONS

1. If a facility has a mammography unit that can image with either Mo anode/Mo filter or Mo anode/Rh filter, which combination should be used for the monthly phantom imaging tests, or should both be used?

2. Usually, the phantom background density (in the middle of the pink wax insert) is 1.2 optical density. If it is 1.5 optical density for this month's test, should corrective action be taken?

3. The compression test reveals that a maximum of 36 pounds can be achieved with the foot pedal. However, when the pedal is released, compression falls to 15 pounds. Is this acceptable?

4. The radiologist at your facility reads many films from outside facilities to provide a second opinion. Should these patients be included in your facility's outcome analysis?

5. A new radiologist joins the staff. Although she has just completed a 1-year fellowship in mammography, she has no continuing medical education credits in mammography. Is she allowed to read mammograms under MQSA regulations?

ANSWERS

1. Only the Mo/Mo combination needs to be tested for monthly phantom images. This image primarily tests AEC stability by recording the mAs needed for the exposure and processor stability to ensure that the same optical density was achieved as for the standard image. Additionally, large changes in kVp and resolution will be noted by recording contrast and speck visibility in the image of the phantom. These factors will not change significantly by replacing the Mo filter with one of Rh so long as a low kVp is used.

2. This is an acceptable optical density for a phantom image sent to the American College of Radiology for mammography accreditation or for establishing the parameters for quarterly phantom imaging. However, if it has already been established that the unit being tested usually produces an image with a background density of 1.2, a 1.5 optical density is out of range and should be corrected. Were the mAs the same as for the preceding month's phantom image? If so, check the daily processor QC. Is the speed index up?

If not, and the phantom image was processed several hours after the daily processor strip was processed, run a second sensitometric strip. Be sure to describe in the QC records the corrective action that was taken.

3. This is a problem commonly experienced when using a unit from one mammography manufacturer. It is not against MQSA regulations. The technologist must reapply compression by hand after releasing the foot pedal.

4. Outcome analysis need not include patients who are not seen at that facility. Because these patients are in the care of the physician who asked for the second opinion, he or she will be responsible for following the patient's outcome.

5. After mammography training in a residency or dedicated fellowship program, the radiologist need not obtain additional continuing medical education credits in mammography for 3 years, at which time 15 additional hours of training must be acquired in the next 3 years.

12

ULTRASOUND

Until recently, ultrasound examinations of the breast have been primarily restricted to differentiating cystic from solid masses. Now, the design of ultrasound equipment has advanced so that diagnostic evaluation of solid masses, in an attempt to differentiate between benign and malignant masses, has become possible (Fig. 12.1). Because of the improvements in ultrasound resolution, a significant proportion of diagnostic examinations of breast masses include ultrasound examination. At many breast centers, core needle biopsies of solid masses are usually performed under ultrasonic guidance. In Japan and Europe (particularly Germany and Italy), ultrasound my be the primary imaging tool for the evaluation of palpable masses. Because palpable masses are usually larger than occult ones they can be diagnosed as malignant or benign with a greater accuracy than is common in the United States.

For patient convenience and to assure continuity of care and integration of mammography and ultrasonography findings, breast ultrasound is usually performed in the mammography suite by radiologists and mammography technologists. This chapter assumes that the reader has no background in ultrasound.

BENIGN VS. MALIGNANT DIAGNOSES

Ultrasound images appear granular and have relatively poor resolution compared with those of other imaging modalities. Like a computed tomography or magnetic resonance image, the ultrasound image represents a slice through tissue rather than a projection of a volume of tissue in a two-dimensional plane. Because the ultrasound slice can be oriented at the discretion of the operator, it can provide a great deal of information about the borders and interiors of suspicious masses. Stravos et al. (listed under "Suggested Readings") describe the many features of malignant breast lesions. Although posterior shadowing (due to attenuation of the sonic beam by the mass) and spiculated, angular, or microlobulated edges are characteristics of malignant lesions, heterogeneous interior echoes and mass shape are less reliable

signs of malignancy. The ability to show these features requires an experienced operator and ultrasound equipment that is designed for examination of the breast. The aim of this chapter is to aid the reader in gaining information about the diagnostic principles of breast ultrasonography and to help the reader select suitable equipment by reviewing some of the basic physics of medical ultrasound.

BACKGROUND PHYSICS AND INSTRUMENTATION

Whereas x-ray mammograms are obtained by the transmission of ionizing radiation through the breast to form a composite shadow of the breast tissue on the image, ultrasound emanations are nonionizing mechanical waves that enter the breast and are reflected from the structures within it, with many returning to the ultrasound transmitter. The depth that the wave travels before it is reflected or scattered back to the transmitting device is calculated by the ultrasound equipment according to the difference in time when the pulse was sent and when it returned. When approximately 100 such waves are sent and reflected back from tissue structures within the breast, an image is formed of a slice through a section of the breast. The mechanical pulsed wave is attenuated by the breast tissue through which it passes so that the returning amplitude of the incident wave is decreased. In fact, some of the returning echoes are 1000 times smaller than they were when transmitted. As a result, the ultrasound equipment must amplify echoes from tissues deeper in the breast more than echoes returned from superficial tissues. This depth dependent amplification is called time gain compensation (TGC) or depth/gain compensation. This attenuation linearly increases with increasing transducer frequency. The resolution of ultrasound images varies with depth and whether the resolution is measured vertically (axial resolution) or horizontally (lateral resolution). In the direction parallel to the direction of travel of the ultrasound beam, resolution of 0.5–1.0 mm depends on the pulse length. In the direction perpendicular to the axial (designated as lateral),

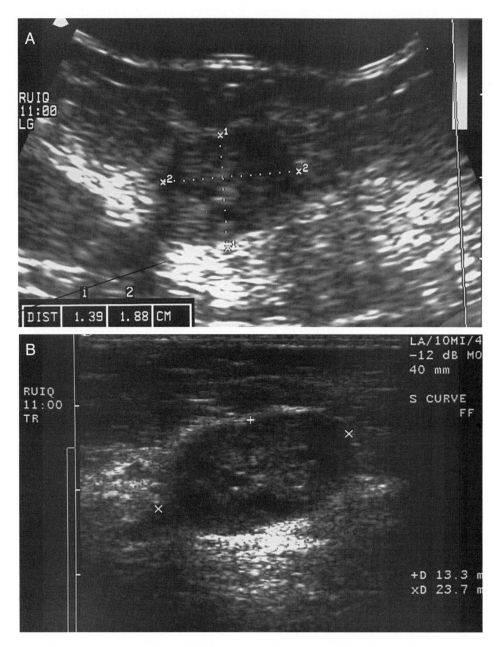

Figure 12.1. Fibroadenoma with interior echoes and posterior enhancement. **A.** Mass imaged with a mechanically oscillated, single crystal, 7.5-MHz transducer. **B.** Mass imaged with an electronically focused 10-MHz linear array. Differences in horizontal caliper measurements are due to poor lateral resolution in image (**A**).

resolution changes with depth, transducer size, and frequency; the technologist can select the depth of interest (focal zone) for each breast. The equipment will then adjust the lateral resolution to 1–2 mm over a 2-cm range; above and below this region, lateral resolution will range from 2 to 4 mm.

The amplitude of the returning pulse is converted into a gray value in the final ultrasound image. An interface between different types of tissue results in a bright echo, represented by a white dot on the image. If the tissue interface is extensive, the dots become a line or boundary of a structure. Pulses of very low amplitude are converted to dark gray dots and are the result of scattering from collections of cells such as fat globules. Masses are represented by collections of these dark gray dots. Because clear fluid does not scatter the ultrasound waves, small cysts have dark, echo-free interiors. The specific gray values assigned to the various ultrasound amplitudes can be changed to increase contrast. Because the ultrasound image is in a digital format, the image can be improved by digital enhancement.

EQUIPMENT

Multipurpose ultrasound equipment costs $150,000–$225,000, but reliable units for breast ultrasound can be purchased for $35,000–$80,000. Because Doppler and color flow measurements have not generally been helpful in diagnosing breast masses smaller than 1.2 cm in diameter, they are not currently considered a necessary component of the ultrasound equipment for a breast center. Two linear or annular array transducers should be purchased. One should operate between 7.5 and 12 MHz and the second from 5 to 6 MHz. The lower frequency transducer will be needed to examine large breasts containing masses located near the chest wall, and the breasts of women with silicone implants. A linear array, which forms a rectangular image, is less expensive than an annular array but requires a fluid offset pad for masses located just under the skin (Fig. 12.2). An annular array forms a wedge-shaped image. Because an annular array has a fluid offset built into the transducer housing, it usually performs well in the evaluation of tissues near the skin. Currently available high frequency annular arrays

are heavy and require a counterbalanced arm to support the wires attaching the transducer to the ultrasound unit. Both annular and linear array transducers consist of many small transducer elements that are pulsed asynchronously to simulate a single element, focused transducer.

Equipment dedicated to ultrasound breast imaging should possess the following essential features:

A magnified image covering only 4 cm in depth;
Focal zones (areas of interest to improve lateral resolution) that can be moved to depths just under the skin;
Electronic calipers that can measure both vertically and horizontally on the same image;
Two alternate contrast options—one for increased latitude and one for increased contrast;
Labeling by means of annotations on the image to identify image locations;
A foot pedal that freezes the image and activates the multiformat camera.

The following features are helpful but not essential:

Icons showing scan planes in the breast;
Edge-sharpening filters;
Persistence, which averages frames to reduce noise in the image;
Cine-loop review—additional storage to save up to 1 second of images so that previous frames can be reviewed to select those most appropriate for printing.

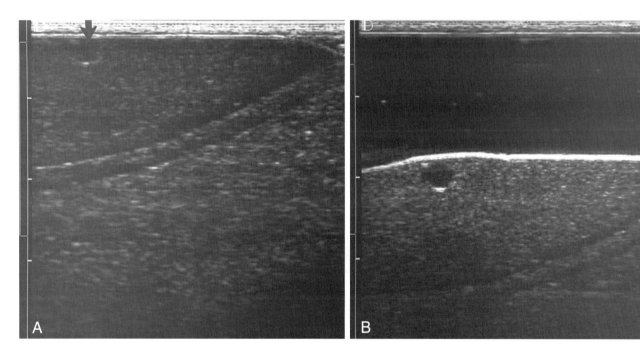

Figure 12.2.   A. A gelatin phantom with a 4-mm "cyst" (*arrow*) embedded under the "skin" of the phantom cannot be well visualized. **B.** When a 2-cm water offset is introduced between phantom and transducer, the "cyst" is clearly seen.

Interior echoes are the result of the small size of the cyst, because scattering from the surrounding tissue artifactually fills in the cyst. Note air bubbles in water offset.

Selected ultrasound images should be recorded on film through the use of a multiformat camera. Polaroid or paper prints are not recommended because of their limited latitude. More expensive, digital methods for making hard copies are available, but they are uneconomical for the relatively small volume of ultrasound examinations that are performed in a breast center. The multiformat camera is attached to the video-out plug located on the back of the ultrasound monitor. Six images can usually be stored on each film.

ULTRASOUND BREAST EXAMINATION

The first step consists of entering the patient's identification and demographic data and the area to be examined on the screen of the ultrasound unit. The patient lays supine and is turned to a position that offers the best evaluation of the breast. For comfort, a pillow or other support is placed under her upper back on the side to be examined. The patient is asked to place her arm, corresponding to the side to be imaged, above her head, which should spread the breast tissue more evenly over the chest wall. Warmed acoustic gel or oil is placed over the area and scanned. The technologist should arrange the patient and ultrasound unit so that the transducer is held in the right hand (if she is right-handed) and adjustments to the ultrasound unit can be made with the left. An initial scan over the area thought to contain the mass will allow the technologist to adjust the focal depth of the image, as well as the TGC, to compensate for attenuation in the breast. Usually, scanning begins with the higher frequency transducer and the gray level map with the greater latitude. If the mass cannot be located in the first 2 cm or if the chest wall cannot be identified, a lower frequency transducer (5–6 MHz) may be needed, in which case focal zone placement, magnification of the image, and TGC will have to be readjusted. Patient position and transducer orientation can also be adjusted to allow the mass to be localized as near the transducer as possible. The parenchyma pattern may contain many fat lobules that simulate masses when imaged transversely. By rotating the transducer 90°, the elongated shape of a fat globule can be readily identified and a mass eliminated.

Once a mass is located, the image is frozen; if it is of diagnostic quality, filming begins. Usually both transverse and longitudinal views through the greatest dimension of the mass are made and then measured with electronic calipers. Occasionally an oblique view can resolve a complex shape (Fig. 12.3). The use of increased contrast will allow interior echoes and mass edges to be examined in more detail. High contrast gray scale maps may be termed "S," "root," or some other designation besides "linear" (Fig. 12.4). Increased contrast will reveal very low amplitude interior echoes which may indicate that the mass is solid rather then cystic. If these echoes float when the breast is tapped, they represent debris in a cyst. If amplification is too high because gain or TGC is excessive, noise will appear at the periphery of the interior of the cyst. Most cysts will have posterior enhancement (Fig. 12.5) because the amplification provided by the TGC is not "used up" by the nonattenuating fluid in the cyst. Although edge enhancement may be useful when evaluating the edges and interiors of masses, it will increase the noise in the image. To reduce noise, frames may be averaged together (persistence) if the transducer can be held stationary during the averaging process.

Although microcalcifications are not routinely imaged ultrasonically, large benign calcifications can be seen because of their bright echoes and posterior shadows. Sometimes the presence of numerous microcalcifications in a mass can be suggested by the presence of both bright interior echoes and streaked posterior shadowing.

Ultrasonically guided core biopsies require the presence of both a radiologist and a technologist. Whereas the radiologist holds the core biopsy gun in his or her dominant hand and ultrasound transducer (which is wrapped in a sterile latex cover) in the alternate hand, the technologist may adjust the ultrasound scanning parameters and documents the position of the needle in the mass with multiformat images (Fig. 12.6). To avoid a pneumothorax, care must be taken to perform the core biopsy parallel rather than perpendicular to the chest wall.

At our institution, experience with ultrasound-guided core biopsies is first gained using a simulated human breast consisting of a raw turkey breast containing stuffed olives. The practicing radiologist who can consistently obtain cores that contain pimento is judged to be sufficiently adept to attempt the biopsy of a true breast mass under appropriate supervision.

QUALITY CONTROL BY THE TECHNOLOGIST

Except for the failure of the electronic caliper, an observant technologist will discover most equipment problems before they are found by routine ultrasound quality control evaluation. To test the calipers, an ultrasound phantom designed for high frequency transducers (small parts phantom) will be needed. Both Nuclear Associates and Gamex manufacture appropriate phantoms, which

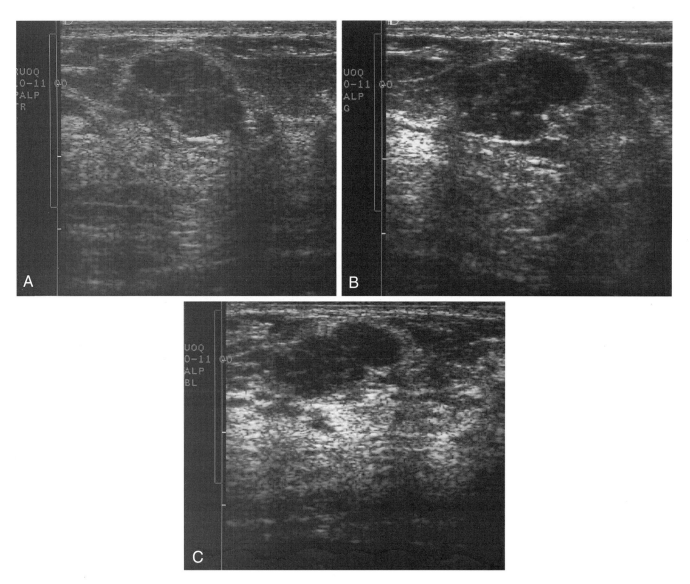

Figure 12.3. Three views of a palpable, lobulated, solid mass. **A.** Transverse view does not image lobulation. **B.** Longitudinal view shows duct (to the left) and possibly three masses. **C.** A single lobulated mass can be seen on the oblique view. If separate masses were present, the higher contrast in image (**C**) would show boundaries between each mass.

cost $2000–$2500. Many small filaments spaced 1–3 cm apart can be imaged and measured to test caliper accuracy in both the horizontal and vertical direction. This test should be accurate to 2 mm. The depth of beam penetration can be tested by maximizing the output power, gain, and TGC (at the bottom of the image) and by setting the focal zone as deep as possible. With the high contrast gray scale map, find the last filament that can be seen with texture around it. The depth of that filament is the penetration depth. For a 7.5- to 12-MHz transducer, the depth should be 3–4 cm. For a 5-MHz transducer, it should be at least 6 cm. If subsequent tests show that this depth has decreased more than 1 cm, the service engineer should be notified. When the penetration test is performed, an image made on the multiformat camera can verify that the camera performance is adequate. Compare the film image with the image on the monitor. Count the number of gray values on the wedge displayed to the side of the ultrasound image (some ultrasound units do not have a gray scale wedge). Do the number of steps seen on the film match those seen on the monitor? (They should match within two steps.) Is contrast similar? Is the background on the film as black as it should be? If the multiformat images are

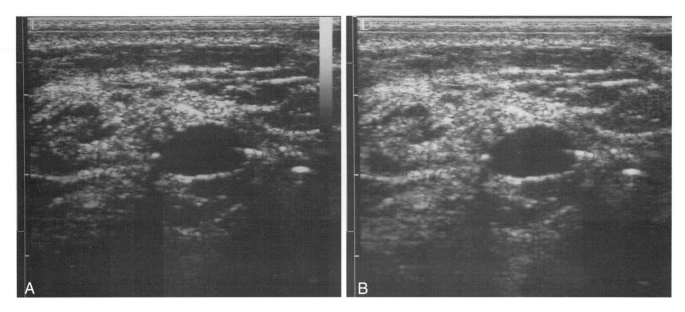

Figure 12.4. **A.** Cyst with linear gray scale map. **B.** Same cyst with increased contrast. Because there are no interior echoes, this is a cystic rather than solid mass. Penetration of the ultrasound beyond 3 cm depth is unsatisfactory.

inferior, either the film processor is underdeveloping or the multiformat camera is out of calibration.

Other tests specific to breast ultrasound can be performed with a raw chicken breast (skin on) and small balloons. The balloons can be filled with water sufficient to create a 1-cm mass, and tied to exclude air. Inserted under the chicken skin, the balloons simulate cysts. To exclude air, the balloons should be coated with acoustic gel before insertion. If the water-filled balloon can be scanned without interior echoes in the half nearest the chicken breast, a linear array is operating correctly. An annular array should image the balloon with no interior echoes. When interior echoes appear throughout the balloon images, the service engineer should examine the equipment and replace any malfunctioning amplification board causing the artifact (see "Problem 3").

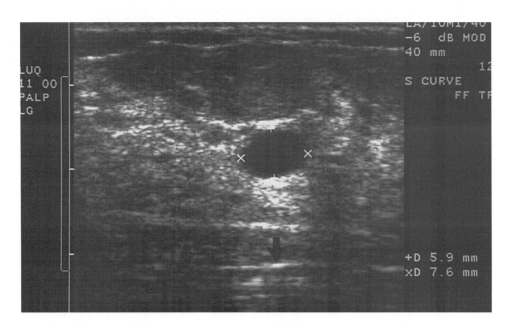

Figure 12.5. Typical appearance of a cyst when imaged with a 10-MHz linear probe. Note posterior enhancement and chest wall (*arrow*).

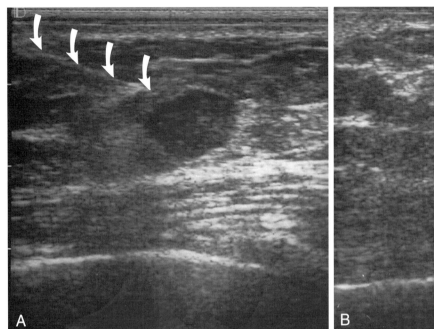
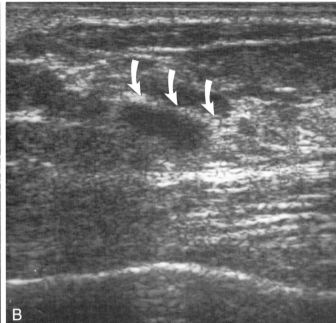

Figure 12.6. Ductal carcinoma with irregular borders and heterogeneous interior echoes. **A.** Prefire before core biopsy. Needle extends from upper left to lesion (*arrows*). **B.** Postfire. Needle now bisects mass (*arrows*).

Although there are many other quality control tests for ultrasound equipment, these simple procedures should suffice for equipment used exclusively for breast examinations.

Suggested Readings

Bassett LW, Kimme-Smith C. Breast sonography. AJR 1991;156:449–455.

This review article contains illustrations of the technical problems encountered during breast ultrasound examinations.

Parker SH, Jobe WE, eds. Percutaneous breast biopsy. New York: Raven, 1993:chapters 10–12.

The technique of breast ultrasound and the ultrasound-guided breast biopsy procedure, both for fine needle aspiration and core biopsy, are described in great detail.

Stravos AT, Thickman D, Rapp CL, Dennis MA, Parker SH, Sisney GA. Solid breast nodules: use of sonography to distinguish between benign and malignant lesions. Radiology 1995;196:123–134.

Malignant and benign ultrasound characteristics of solid masses are described. In a review of 750 cases of solid masses, ultrasonography findings are compared with biopsy results.

PROBLEM 1

A palpable mass is not visible on mammography (*left*) until marked with a BB and imaged with the breast rotated slightly (*right*). Is the second view sufficient for diagnosis?

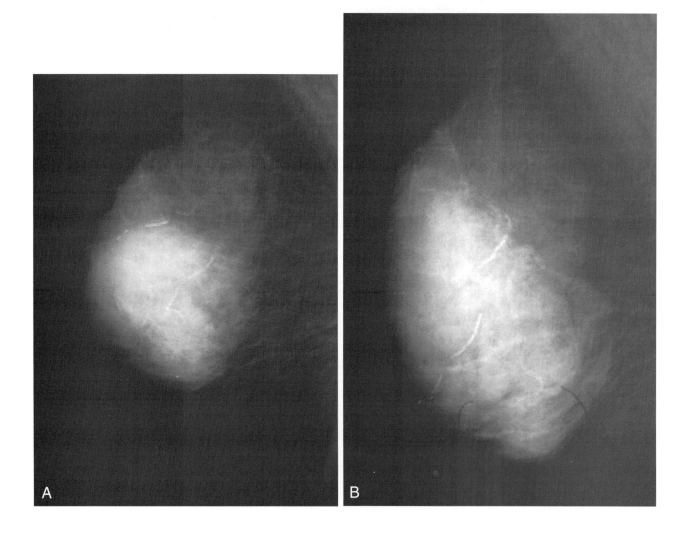

SOLUTION 1

No. Ultrasound examination reveals a highly suspicious solid mass. The glandular tissue surrounding the mass makes diagnosis with mammography difficult.

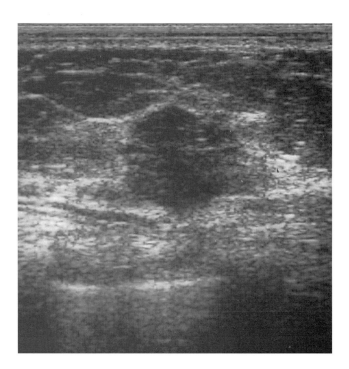

PROBLEM 2

What could have happened to this ultrasound image? Should the transducer be sent back to the manufacturer as defective?

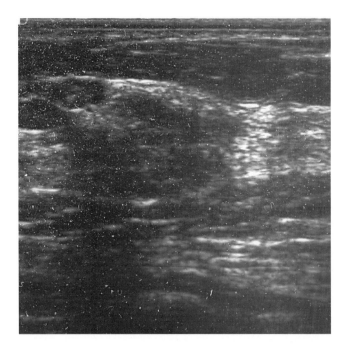

SOLUTION 2

No. The multiformat camera has been in storage and was attached to the ultrasound unit without any maintenance. As a result, dust on the surface of the glass in front of the film was recorded along with the ultrasound image.

PROBLEM 3

Interior echoes in this cystic appearing mass are faint. Are they real or due to scattering from the surrounding tissue?

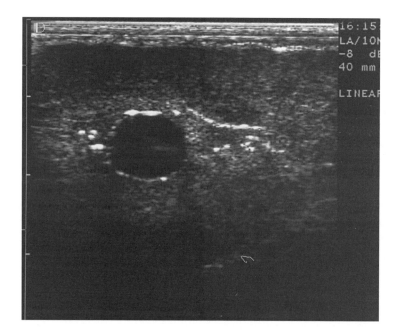

SOLUTION 3

They are real. By changing the contrast, the structure of the echoes can be appreciated.

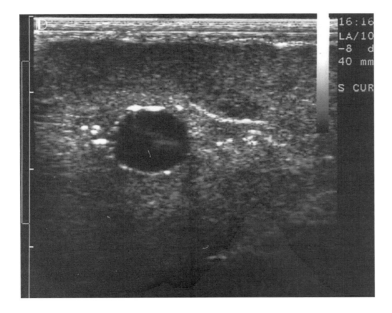

PROBLEM 4

This palpable mass lies deep against the chest wall. What might improve our ability to decide on a biopsy? (Note information about contrast, focal zone, and transducer frequency has been cropped in this photograph.)

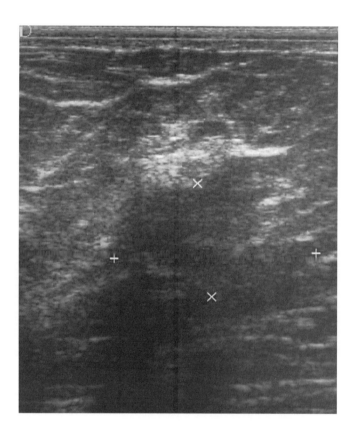

SOLUTION 4

Because the mass is 3 cm deep, the 10-MHz probe cannot image the posterior edge of the mass. First move the focal zone as deep as possible. If this does not improve the image, change to a 5-MHz transducer.

PROBLEM 5

There is a gray streak down the middle of this ultrasound image (*arrows*). There is no apparent breast structure to cause this change; what could cause it?

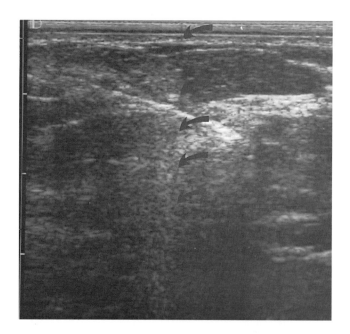

SOLUTION 5

A transducer element in the linear array is missing or firing at a lower intensity. This causes a discontinuity in the image. The transducer should be returned to the manufacturer.

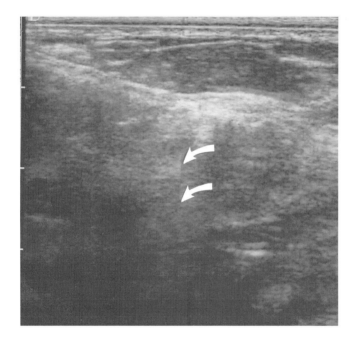

QUESTIONS

1. Toward the end of breast ultrasound examinations, you notice that it is difficult to penetrate the breast and that there are numerous shadows (black streaks) on all images. When you begin a new examination, these problems are not present. What caused the problems?

2. For some breasts the annular array leaves a streak of horizontal bright echoes at about 3.5 cm depth. What causes this artifact?

3. One radiologist prefers to have the ultrasound exam- ination room lights dim, whereas another, who is not as well acquainted with the controls of the ultrasound unit, requires more illumination. The multiformat camera images of the latter are poor, chiefly because the gain of the image is high so that cysts fill in. How could turning up the room lights affect the multiformat images?

4. The vertical caliper accuracy quality assurance test is correct, but for the horizontal caliper accuracy test, an annular array transducer measures a 3-cm space as 3.3 cm. Is this acceptable? What factors could cause this error?

ANSWERS

1. The acoustic gel coating the breast has probably become too thin, and scanning is taking place with insufficient coupling. In this case, air has been trapped between the transducer and skin. Because the ultrasound wave is reflected off of these small pockets of air, it does not penetrate the breast, leaving black areas where no signals return.

2. The annular array is located 3–4 cm behind the membrane that rests on the breasts. When scanning a breast with less attenuation than usual (or when gain is very high), echoes from the reverberation between the transducer and the membrane are mapped as though they were as deep in the breast as the distance between the membrane and the transducer. Because the annular array usually would not penetrate so deeply, these reverberations will not usually be seen.

3. When scanning in a well lighted room, the ultrasound monitor appears dark, and increased TGC or gain will be needed to see to the desired depth in the breast. Because the multiformat camera is calibrated with an ultrasound image made in a dimly lighted room, bright echoes will be saturated if the gain is set inappropriately high. Once the less experienced radiologist has made initial adjustments in scanning parameters, the room lights should be dimmed to allow the ultrasound image to be evaluated under more optimal ambient lighting conditions.

4. Vertical caliper accuracy depends on the velocity of sound calibration in the ultrasound unit. Once it is found to be accurate during acceptance testing, it is likely to remain accurate unless major changes are made in the ultrasound equipment or computer software. For linear arrays, horizontal caliper accuracy depends on the spacing between transducer elements and is unlikely to change after acceptance testing for these transducers. However, annular arrays are rotated by a motor to sweep the beam across the breast. If this motor moves too slowly or irregularly, horizontal distance calibration will be affected. The transducer should be returned to the manufacturer for repair, because a 3-mm error is unacceptable.

13

DIGITAL MAMMOGRAPHY

Users are generally enthusiastic about digital stereotactic breast biopsy systems because they are convenient to use, permit manipulation of image contrast after the x-ray exposure, and provide an image more speedily than a standard film processor.

However, the extension of this digital technology to a whole breast digital mammography system will require overcoming certain technological problems. Prototype whole breast digital systems are being tested in several breast imaging centers, and commercial systems will be available after Food and Drug Administration approval. Because they are expected to be much more expensive than current screen/film systems, what added benefits do they offer to justify the increased cost? Will they be capable of detecting cancer earlier, particularly in dense, glandular breasts, than is currently possible? Will we find, as we did with dedicated breast ultrasound, that the additional lesions that are detected are usually benign and that the use of the new equipment only increases the number of benign biopsies? Despite their use of Rh and W anodes, current mammography units cannot be relied on to detect small cancers in glandular breasts because of insufficient contrast. Enhancement of contrast by digital mammography systems should help to alleviate this problem (Fig. 13.1). Another benefit of whole breast digital mammography, and one that is featured by digital

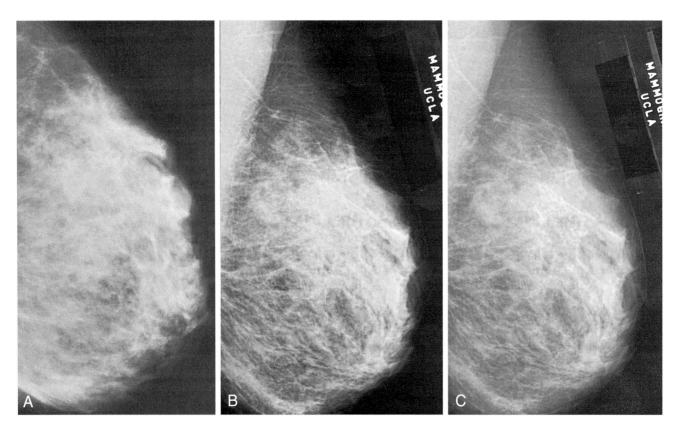

Figure 13.1. A dense breast imaged with screen/film (**A**) and computed radiography (**B**) using a photostimulable plate read by a laser. Contrast enhancement saturates glandular tissue. **C.** Same image as **B** but with a linear characteristic (gray scale) curve and edge enhancement to help restore image sharpness lost by the 100-micron pixel size of the laser read-out.

breast biopsy units, is the speed with which the digital image is obtained. Because cassettes do not have to be inserted and removed from the cassette tunnel, because poor positioning can be corrected more quickly, and because overexposure can be corrected during image processing, we should expect to double the number of patients that can be screened by one unit in a given period.

In the future, when many large imaging centers will be filmless, digital mammography will be in their armamentarium to avoid storage and retrieval of films. As soon as this new equipment has been shown to be reliable, it will be used in mobile mammography vans and at remote centers where the images can be stored and read later or transmitted electronically to the parent center for immediate review. The quality of digital mammography equipment can be expected to be more reliable than that of standard mammography equipment because the exposure latitude will be greater and film processing problems will have been eliminated.

Many academic centers are designing computer-aided diagnostic equipment to automatically signal the presence of a suspicious breast lesion or to predict whether it is malignant (computer-aided detection). This innovative equipment is being tested on digitized film mammograms. With the availability of digital mammograms, computer-aided detection may augment our ability to detect cancer. Another benefit of digital mammography may be increased ease of localizing lesions for needle placement or additional views. Equipment may be devised that will automatically move a needle or compression paddle above the location of the lesion. To obtain a magnified image, digital mammography units of the future may even be able to change focal spots and digital resolution automatically rather than requiring the breast to be placed on a platform above the film cassette.

DIGITAL EQUIPMENT

Unlike computed radiography, where an imaging plate is placed in a cassette, exposed, and then inserted into a reader, digital mammography features a built-in image receptor that is read immediately after the x-ray exposure. Current systems use a fluorescent material, such as cesium iodide, to convert x-rays to light photons. The light photons are detected by solid state detectors, usually charge coupled devices or amorphous silicon, which convert them to electrons. The number of electrons represents the intensity of the signal or the amount of x-rays passing through the breast. The image receptor resolution determines the overall system resolution so long as the fluorescent material does not degrade the in-

herent resolution represented by the magnification factor and the number and size of pixels in the solid state detector. Most digital mammography systems can be expected to have pixels representing about 50 microns each at the location of the breast.

Several methods are used by different manufacturers to transmit the light photons to the solid state detectors. Some use fiberoptic cabling, whereas another directly coats the detector with the fluorescent material. These detectors may be arranged in an array of up to 12 elements, each containing more than 1000 elements on a side; they are placed close together to make a large area detector that can image the whole breast. In one digital unit with a slot system, the high voltage generator and the movement of the slot across the breast are synchronized.

A digital mammography unit is identical to a screen/film unit except for the image recording system. Patient positioning is similar to that for a film system. Automatic exposure control depends primarily on compressed breast thickness. Although small differences in exposure will not affect image quality, an attempt to lower the dose to the patient by inappropriately decreasing the exposure will result in excessive noise that could obscure calcifications (see "Problem 3" in Chapter 4). To prevent this, the manufacturer's exposure recommendations should be carefully followed.

Once an exposure has been made, an image appears on the acquisition workstation, allowing the technologist to check the positioning. In general, resolution of the image at this workstation will not be as high as at the display workstation, which is used by the radiologist for diagnostic evaluation of the images. Although initially most centers will probably elect to make a hard copy of the image through the use of a laser printer whose resolution will be matched to the resolution of the digital mammography unit, the image will be stored on a disk for evaluation at any time.

The display workstation can be expected to evolve from those now available that only display multiple images, zoom on suspicious areas, and enhance by window and level operations.

DIGITAL TECHNIQUE

The patient's name and medical identification number are entered by the technologist on the acquisition workstation just as is done for computed tomography, magnetic resonance imaging, and ultrasound examinations. The patient is positioned and the breast compressed as usual. The equipment displays the kVp and mAs after the exposure. Most units will require a technique between 28 and 33 kVp. Digital enhancement permits restoration of any subject contrast that might have been lost by imaging at such a high kVp. The higher kVp exposure improves the signal-to-noise ratio without increasing the dose as much as it would have been increased at a lower kVp exposure. Once the exposure is made, the image appears on the acquisition workstation, usually within 10 seconds. If a repeat exposure is needed, it can be obtained immediately. The radiologist can review the examination at the display workstation while the patient is still at the facility, or the radiologist can review the images later.

Because images are automatically stored on an optical disk, no hard copies are needed unless the radiologist prefers them or the images must be sent to another facility. In this case, the technologist or an image specialist reviews the images on the display workstation and enhances them appropriately for printing. Printing is ac-

complished by using methods similar to those used for printing images of computed tomography and magnetic resonance imaging scans (Fig. 13.2).

Before the images are permanently stored, the data are compressed to occupy less storage space. Most compression techniques currently used for mammography do not affect image quality. In the future, so many more mammograms will be stored that some minor information may be lost, but the overall diagnostic content should remain the same.

Contrast enhancement of digital mammograms is similar to that of computed radiographic or magnetic resonance images. Once the type of tissue that predominates has been identified, the contrast can be manipulated by changing the latitude of the image. A very glandular (BI RADS category 4) breast (Fig. 13.3) requires different enhancement from that required for a fatty breast (BI RADS category 1) (Fig. 13.4). Although enhancement of the edges of structures in the breast should aid in the de-

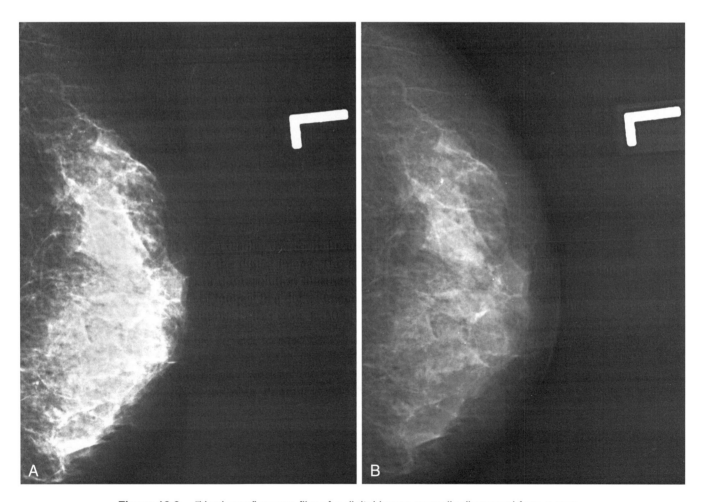

Figure 13.2. "Hard copy" means film of a digital image normally diagnosed from a monitor (**A**). When printed, both the characteristic curve and the contrast must be modified (**B**).

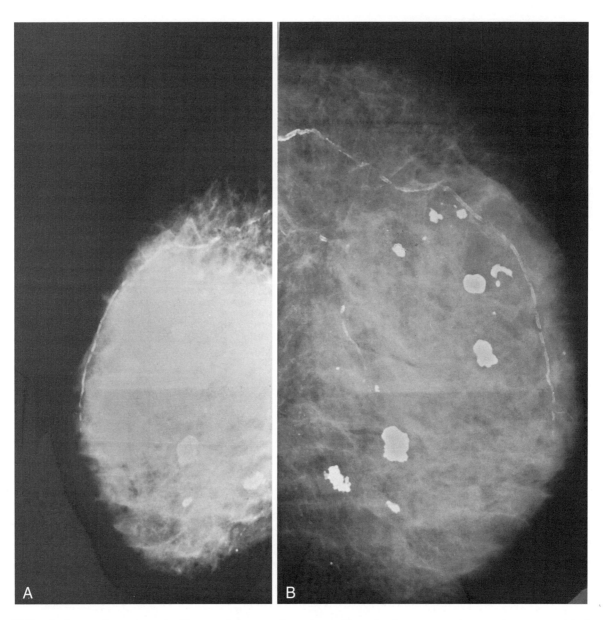

Figure 13.3. **A.** A very dense breast with no enhancement to the digital image (called a "raw" image). **B.** Same breast (repositioned) after gray scale mapping appropriate for a BI RADS category 4 breast (magnified 1.2×).

tection of microcalcifications, it may cause distortion as well. Subtle calcifications, which may appear to have fuzzy borders on conventional film images, may appear brighter and sharper when edge enhanced (Fig. 13.5).

QUALITY CONTROL

When all mammography equipment has become digital, the technologists will be delighted that they no longer have to perform daily processor sensitometric testing, fixer clearance tests, or darkroom fog tests. However, because most facilities will have a combination of digital and screen/film units for several transition years, these tests cannot be immediately discontinued. Until the reliability of digital units has been firmly established, daily or weekly imaging of a phantom will be required. Research on the automated interpretation of these phantom images may eventually lead to the technologist being relieved of the burdens of densitometric evaluation and plotting target visibility. Instead, these functions would be performed by the acquisition workstation using computer programs to analyze the phantom images. The digital mammography unit, like screen/film units,

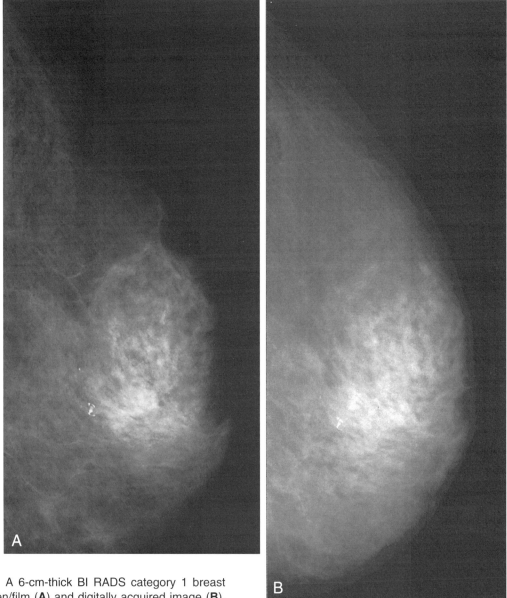

Figure 13.4. A 6-cm-thick BI RADS category 1 breast seen on screen/film (**A**) and digitally acquired image (**B**).

will require testing for artifacts but at more frequent intervals. This will probably consist of imaging a screen/film contact mesh or plastic sheets to create a regular pattern against which artifacts will be recognizable. Test of breast compression will still be needed. Retake analysis will be automatic, because the number of additional images will be recorded by the acquisition workstation and the reason for the repeated exposure may be stored.

The physicist will have additional responsibilities when performing acceptance testing and surveying the digital unit. In addition to the usual tests performed on the generator, focal spot, and mechanical components of a mammography unit, the physicist will need to assess the image receptor for artifacts and interdetector irregularities. Instead of testing the automatic exposure control (or built-in technique chart) for optical density variations, the physicist will have to estimate signal-to-noise ratio at the preassigned techniques. This can best be achieved by adding Lucite to a standardized phantom, such as the American College of Radiology mammography accreditation phantom, to determine if the technique prescribed for each breast thickness allows postenhancement visualization of the appropriate number of targets in the phantom. However, physicists will be pleased to note that they will not have to test screen/film cassettes for uniformity.

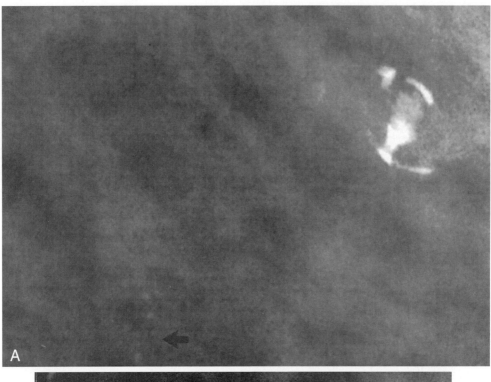

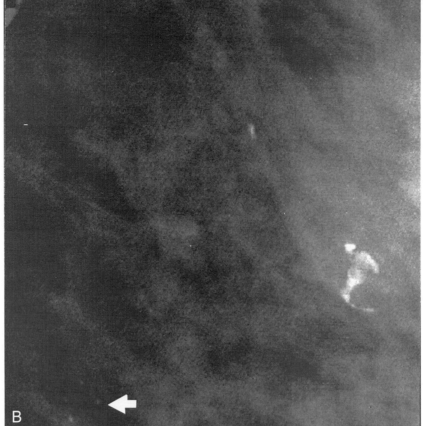

Figure 13.5. Detail of calcifications in Figure 13.4 seen on screen/film (**A**) and digitally acquired image (**B**).

The introduction of digital mammography to a clinical situation may be easier than had formerly been predicted because, having no processor-related problems, they are expected to be more reliable than screen/film systems. The expected increased reliability may lead to the easing of regulations and quality control procedures that have burdened technologists and physicists since 1994. In addition, the capability of contrast manipulation may result in a better imaging tool than current screen/film mammography systems.

Suggested Readings

Rougeot H. Direct x-ray conversion processes. In: Hendee WR, Trueblood JH, eds. Digital imaging. American Association of Physicists in Medicine Summer School Proceedings 22. Madison WI: Medical Physics Publishing, 1993.

This technical article describes one technique used for digital mammography. The reader will understand some of the design decisions used for a highly successful system.

Shtern F. Digital mammography and related technologies: a perspective from the National Cancer Institute. Radiology 1992;183:629–630.

This short article describes the clinical benefits that may result from digital mammography.

Yaffe MJ. Digital mammography. In: Haus AG, Yaffe MJ, eds. Syllabus: a categorical course in physics. Technical aspects of breast imaging, Radiological Society of North America 80th Annual Meeting, Nov 27–Dec 2, 1994.

The problems inherent in designing a digital system for mammography are surveyed. Although technical, it is clearly written. The author is responsible for initiating the design of most current digital mammography systems.

PROBLEM 1

The digital mammogram (**A**) has a cluster of calcifications (*arrow*). When we zoom to that region of interest (**B**), enhancement has artifactually created other calcifications. How can these artifacts be avoided?

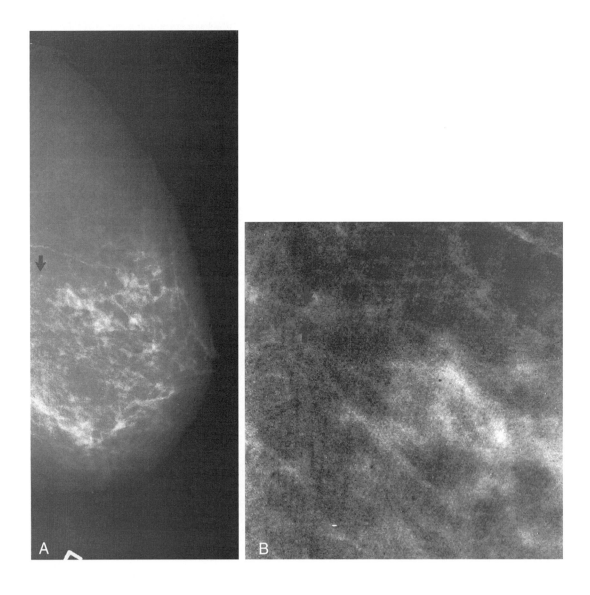

SOLUTION 1

Reduce the contrast in the region of interest. Initially, the radiologist and technologist may experience some frustration while selecting the correct level of contrast for digital mammograms. The dark lines are the result of electronic noise that has been enhanced along with the contrast.

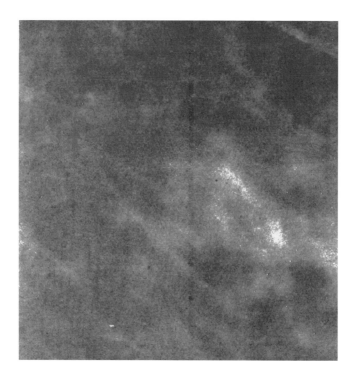

PROBLEM 2

How can the calcifications distributed throughout this digital mammogram be evaluated more effectively?

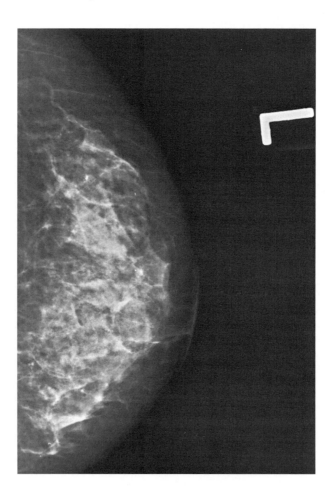

SOLUTION 2

By applying an edge enhancement filter without increasing contrast. This processing will only be successful if the exposure was sufficiently high to ensure a good signal-to-noise ratio.

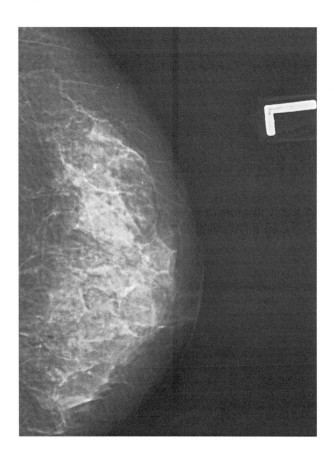

PROBLEM 3

How would you process this image so the skin line would be visible and dense glandular tissue have greater contrast?

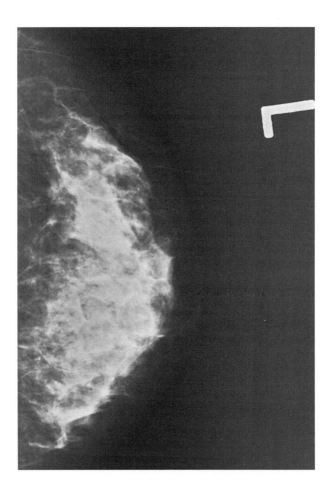

SOLUTION 3

Change the optical density of the glandular tissue to a darker shade of gray, and reduce overall contrast to improve image latitude.

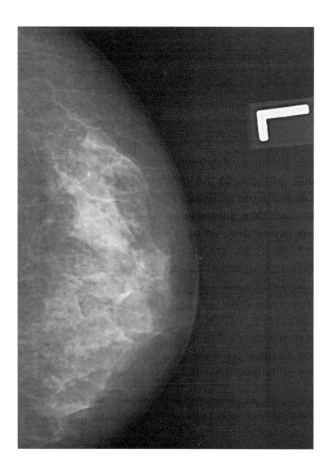

PROBLEM 4

Why are these calcifications visible in this zoomed image when they were not visible in the raw image (Fig. 13.3*A*)?

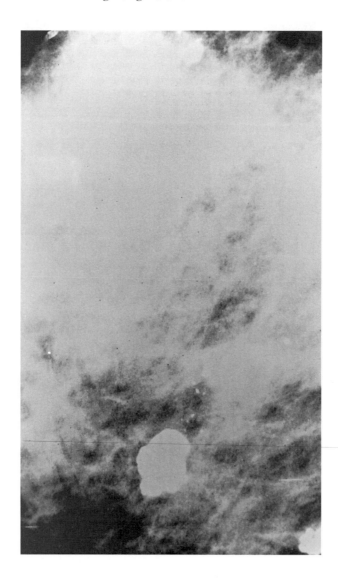

SOLUTION 4

Monitors cannot display the entire breast with the same spatial resolution that is available in the digital image. The resolution shown in Figure 3A is one-quarter that of the resolution illustrated under "Problem 4." When we zoom on a region of interest in a digital image, we are viewing the image at a much higher resolution; in this case, at 50 microns instead of 200 microns.

QUESTIONS

1. Because the display workstation can optically magnify clusters of microcalcifications in digital mammograms, is there any reason to obtain magnification mammograms?

2. Why can't the noise in an underexposed mammogram be smoothed by image processing?

3. Because digital mammography can use higher kVp (the lower subject contrast can be enhanced by image processing), penetration is increased. Because digital mammography has greater latitude, the breast does not have to be of uniform thickness. Why then does the breast require compression during digital mammography?

4. Last year a woman whose compressed breast thickness was 4.5 cm received 95 mrad mean glandular dose for a craniocaudal screen/film mammogram. This year she received 170 mrad for the same view obtained with a digital unit. Is this acceptable?

ANSWERS

1. An optically magnified image will be as blurred as the unmagnified image. Although it will be bigger, it will contain no more information about the edges and shape of the microcalcifications than the image viewed without optical magnification.

2. Noise can be made less noticeable by averaging the optical density values of adjacent pixels. However, this procedure also blurs the signal along with the noise, so no increase in information will result.

3. For the same reasons that screen/film imaging benefits from compression: to reduce scatter and mean glandular dose and to spread the tissue so there are fewer overlapping structures.

4. Yes, because the higher dose may represent a more informative mammogram. Furthermore, because her breast was compressed to 4.5 cm, we can compare the doses with those of the American College of Radiology mammography accreditation phantom. The mean glandular dose received from the digital unit was below state and national recommended limits.

REVIEW QUESTIONS AND ANSWERS

QUESTIONS

1. Which developer chemical controls the low optical density development?
   a. hydroquinone
   b. bromide
   c. sulfites
   d. phenidone

2. Which statements are true about starter used in film processors?
   a. It contains bromides.
   b. It must be added to the developer tank at the start of each day to compensate for overnight developer oxidation.
   c. It is part of the fixer replenishment system.
   d. It is only necessary in low volume practices.

3. Many mammography tubes are tilted to improve _____.
   a. the heel effect
   b. tube output
   c. focal spot size (length)
   d. off-focus radiation

4. The density steps ($+2$, $+1$, 0, -1, -2) in an automatic exposure control for mammography should differ from each other by _____.
   a. 20–30%
   b. 15–20%
   c. 10–15%
   d. 5–10%

5. Base + fog of 0.25 could not be caused by _____.
   a. high temperature in the film storage area
   b. developer temperature above 100°F
   c. poor wall shielding in the film storage area
   d. oxidized developer

6. Contrast (film gradient) for mammography film reaches its maximum near what optical density?
   a. 0.2–0.6
   b. 0.6–1.0

   c. 1.0–1.4
   d. 1.4–1.8
   e. above 1.8

7. An "ortho" film means it is _____.
   a. used to image bones
   b. sensitive to green light
   c. has a reciprocity failure rate below 5%
   d. double-sided

8. Compression paddles should be _____.
   a. rounded at the chest wall to prevent injury to the patient
   b. fireproof
   c. transparent
   d. at least 3 mm thick

9. Grid ratio for mammography ranges from _____.
   a. 3.5:1 to 5:1
   b. 5:1 to 8.5:1
   c. 8.5:1 to 11:1
   d. none of the above

10. If a mammography grid designed for a 50-cm source-to-image unit is used on a 60-cm source-to-image unit, then _____.
    a. dose will increase
    b. there is no problem with this substitution
    c. edges (right and left) of the film will be lighter than the center
    d. the heel effect will be increased by grid cut-off

11. MQSA requires that kVp should be accurate within _____.
    a. 1.5 kVp
    b. 1%
    c. 2.5 kVp
    d. 2%

12. The QA technologist should image the American College of Radiology phantom _____.
    a. daily
    b. weekly

225

c. monthly
d. semiannually

13. For digital stereotactic units, what difference in the American College of Radiology phantom image (compared with film) is true?
   a. Less exposure is needed.
   b. All five masses are visible.
   c. Four or more clusters of calcifications are visible.
   d. The heel effect makes only half the phantom visible.

14. Window and level refer to _____.
   a. an operation that changes the contrast in digital images
   b. the collimation and position of the digital receptor in the field of view
   c. the lens size and position in the digital camera
   d. the number of bits per pixel in a digital image

15. TGC in breast ultrasound refers to _____.
   a. increasing amplification with depth
   b. temperature gain compensation
   c. focusing deeper to improve penetration
   d. tomosynthetic geocystic lesions

16. Breast ultrasound cannot be used for _____.
   a. needle biopsies
   b. microcalcification localization
   c. lactating women
   d. women younger than 30

17. As kVp and HVL increase, the conversion factor for calculating mean glandular dose _____.
   a. decreases
   b. stays the same
   c. increases

18. As breast thickness increases by 1 cm, exposure _____ while the mean glandular conversion factor _____.
   a. doubles/increases
   b. doubles/decreases
   c. increases 50%/increases
   d. increases 50%/stays the same
   e. increases 50%/decreases

19. What dose reducing method is most effective?
   a. increase kVp or use a Rh anode/Rh filter
   b. increase compression

c. increase processing temperature
d. use extended processing
e. reduce optical density from 1.6 to 1.4

20. A level 1 Mammography Quality Standards Act finding _____.
   a. must be corrected by the next inspection
   b. must be corrected within 1 month of inspection by stating corrective action taken
   c. will cause your facility not to be certified if not corrected immediately

21. Fixed grids are not recommended for new mammography equipment because _____.
   a. they do not reciprocate
   b. the interspace material hardens the x-ray beam, reducing contrast
   c. they increase dose to the patient
   d. they are easily damaged
   e. they are too expensive

22. The row of four masses in the American College of Radiology mammography phantom should be aligned with the _____.
   a. right-hand side
   b. left-hand side
   c. chest wall
   d. top of the film (anode side)

23. How often is darkroom fog measured?
   a. every 6 months
   b. monthly
   c. weekly
   d. daily

24. A "daylight" processor still requires a darkroom at the facility where it is located because _____.
   a. film canisters must be loaded in a darkroom
   b. sensitometric strips must be exposed
   c. unexposed film must be stored in a darkroom
   d. film jams must be corrected in a darkroom
   e. a darkroom is not needed

25. The thicker the screen, the _____ the speed of the system and the _____ the resolution of the resulting image.
   a. slower/higher
   b. slower/lower
   c. faster/higher
   d. faster/lower

26. Dye in the screens _____.
    a. converts the blue emission to green
    b. controls the spreading of light photons
    c. gives mammograms the blue base + fog color
    d. allows us to use a red safe light in the darkroom

27. Light sensitometry tests the _____ combination.
    a. screen/film
    b. film/processor
    c. screen/film/processor
    d. screen/film/processor/darkroom
    e. film/processor/darkroom

28. Film reciprocity law failure affects _____.
    a. contrast
    b. speed
    c. base + fog
    d. maximum optical density

29. Latent image fading results when _____.
    a. long exposures are needed
    b. very short immersion times in the processor occur
    c. processing exposed film is delayed significantly
    d. unexposed film is stored too long

30. Mammography film, compared with film used for chest radiography, is _____.
    a. slower, with greater latitude
    b. single-sided with more contrast
    c. has a lower base + fog and lower resolution
    d. double-sided with greater resolution

31. Where is the automatic exposure sensor located on mammography units?
    a. above the grid
    b. between the grid and the screen/film cassette
    c. below the screen/film cassette
    d. wherever the technologist positions it

32. Where should the automatic exposure sensor be positioned when imaging a breast containing a silicone implant?
    a. at the chest wall
    b. at the nipple
    c. in the middle of the breast so that the silicone implant covers it
    d. does not matter because a manual exposure is needed

33. A magnification view of a section of the breast requires that we change the _____.
    a. source-to-image distance
    b. type of screen/film receptor
    c. focal spot
    d. compression paddle
    e. grid ratio

34. Core biopsies of the breast are performed with what gauge needle?
    a. 14
    b. 18
    c. 20
    d. 22

35. Specimen imaging cannot be performed on which of the following imaging devices?
    a. mammography unit with small focal spot
    b. prone stereotactic unit
    c. faxitron (a stand-alone small x-ray source)
    d. 10-MHz ultrasound unit

36. One benefit of prone stereotactic biopsy is _____.
    a. breast compression need not be so aggressive
    b. the radiologist can be seated throughout the procedure
    c. if the patient faints, she won't fall
    d. digital receptors are available

37. What method of dose reduction will not affect contrast?
    a. increased compression
    b. faster screen/film system
    c. extended processing
    d. increased kVp
    e. use of a Rh/Rh combination anode/filter

38. A woman whose breasts can be compressed to 6 cm would be likely to receive about what mean glandular dose from a screening examination if a Mo anode/Mo filter were used?
    a. 300 mrad
    b. 600 mrad
    c. 1 rad
    d. 2 rad

39. Why is it important to have a high maximum optical density on mammography films?
    a. to eliminate ambient light when using high intensity mammography viewers

b. to increase the apparent contrast in the film

c. so that the skin line can be seen without hot lighting

d. not an important attribute of mammography film, which is why it is not plotted during quality control

40. If the speed point varies by a certain amount, the film producing that measurement cannot be used. What is the amount of variation?
    a. 0.15 optical density
    b. 15% variation from the set speed point optical density
    c. 0.10 optical density
    d. 10% variation from the set speed point optical density

41. What factor is most important for good resolution in mammography?
    a. focal spot size
    b. location of lesion in breast
    c. screen speed
    d. grid or no grid
    e. compression

42. Limiting resolution (with a high contrast phantom) for mammography is about _____.
    a. 2 line pairs/mm
    b. 8 line pairs/mm
    c. 15 line pairs/mm
    d. 20 line pairs/mm

43. From the chest wall to the nipple, resolution _____.
    a. improves
    b. stays the same
    c. worsens

44. Magnification uses a smaller focal spot because _____.
    a. less breast is imaged
    b. a grid is not used
    c. blur is magnified too
    d. the higher kVp allows fewer mAs to be used

45. The smaller the focal spot, the _____.
    a. lower the mAs
    b. lower the mA
    c. higher the mA
    d. higher the kVp
    e. lower the dose

46. Whole breast digital mammography will not change (compared with screen/film mammography) the _____.
    a. kVp used
    b. compression needed
    c. grid used
    d. quality control procedures

47. Breast ultrasound resolution is about:
    a. 3 line pairs/cm
    b. 1 line pair/mm
    c. 3 line pairs/mm
    d. 5 line pairs/mm

48. A stand-off pad may be necessary for breast ultrasound if _____.
    a. an annular array is used
    b. the mass is less than 1 cm deep
    c. the mass is more than 3 cm deep
    d. the patient's breasts are very glandular

49. Patients are advised not to use deodorant before an examination because _____.
    a. residue is left on the breast support system, which is not hygienic
    b. it will increase the exposure needed
    c. it may cause calcification-like artifacts on the mammograms
    d. it can interact with the plastic in the compression paddle, causing pitting

50. By imaging with a Rh anode/Rh filter instead of a Mo/Mo combination, the mean keV is _____.
    a. lowered 3 keV
    b. stays the same; the peak changes
    c. raised 3 keV
    d. raised 5 keV

ANSWERS

1. d. Chapter 9, "Chemistry," paragraph 2

2. a. Chapter 9, "Chemistry," paragraph 3

3. See Figure 6.1.

4. c. Chapter 5, last sentence before "AEC Exposure Termination"

5. d. Chapter 9, "Chemistry," paragraph 3 and your knowledge that a and c could cause fogging; b can be eliminated by information in Chapter 9, "Chemistry," next-to-last paragraph

6. e. See Figure 8.3 and realize why darker films are recommended.

7. b. Chapter 8, "Film," paragraph 1

8. c. Figures 3.1 and 3.4 show how useful it is for the technologist to be able to see the positioned breast through the compression paddle; answer a would prevent pulling the breast away from the chest wall.

9. a. Chapter 7, "Grids," paragraph 1

10. c. This information can be inferred from Chapter 7, "Grids," paragraph 2 but is not explicitly stated. If the SID is not matched to the grid focusing, grid cut-off will occur at each side because the grid is focused at 50 cm while, in fact, the SID is 60 cm.

11. a. The American College of Radiology recommendation is 5% of the kVp tested, although it is not covered in the workbook.

12. c. Chapter 11, "Technologist's Quality Assurance," paragraph 3

13. c. Chapter 4, "Problem 3"

14. a. Chapter 13, "Digital Technique," paragraph 4

15. a. Chapter 12, "Background Physics and Instrumentation," paragraph 1

16. b. Chapter 12, "Ultrasound Breast Examination," paragraph 3

17. c. See Table 10.1

18. b. See Table 10.1

19. b. If tolerated, otherwise d or c (a and e affect image quality); Chapter 10, "Mammography Equipment: Effect on Dose," next-to-last paragraph

20. c. Chapter 11, "MQSA Inspection," paragraph 1

21. a and b. The workbook does not give a reason. By not reciprocating, small grid lines are left on the mammogram that distract the viewer. Also, the interspace material is aluminum, not carbon fibers, so contrast is degraded. Answers c and d are also correct but are not the reason for a lack of recommendation.

22. c. Note orientation and heel effect (which shows where the chest wall is located) in "Problem 1."

23. a. Chapter 11, "Technologist's Quality Assurance," paragraph 6

24. a and b. Chapter 11, "Technologist's Quality Assurance," paragraph 1

25. d. Chapter 8, "Screens," paragraph 3

26. b. Chapter 8, "Screens," paragraphs 1 and 2

27. e. The screen is not tested by light sensitometry, but the rest of the imaging chain is tested.

28. b. Chapter 8, "Film Reciprocity Law Failure"

29. c. Chapter 8, "Latent Image Fading"

30. b. Chapter 8, "Film," paragraph 1

31. c. Figure 5.1

32. d. Chapter 5, "Problem 3"

33. c. Chapter 6, "Focal Spot Size and SID"

34. a. Figure 4.7

35. d. Chapter 12, "Background Physics and Instrumentation," end of paragraph 1; poor resolution prevents ultrasound from being used for specimen imaging

36. c. Chapter 4, "Dedicated Prone Stereotactic Core Breast Biopsy"

37. b. Contrast is increased for answers a and c and decreased for d and e. Of course, some faster screen/film systems have increased contrast, but increased speed is usually achieved by making the screen thicker, which does not affect contrast.

38. c. Chapter 10, "Mammography Equipment: Effect on Dose," paragraph 6. It is implied that exposure doubles for each centimeter of breast thickness. If a 4-cm breast receives about 1.07 R, then a 6-cm breast would receive four times that amount (4.28 R), and two views would require 8.56 R. Using Table 10.1, the conversion factor is between 0.11 and 0.12; mean glandular dose is nearly 1 rad.

39. b. Although average gradient does not change as maximum optical density increases, the apparent contrast increases because blacks are blacker.

40. a. The answer is found in the American College of Radiology quality control manual.

41. a. Chapter 6, "Focal Spot Size and SID," paragraph 1; screen speed will not degrade resolution as much as a large focal spot

42. c. Figure 6.4, curve for M = 1.08

43. a. Figure 6.3

44. c. Chapter 6, "Focal Spot Size and SID," paragraph 1

45. b. Chapter 6, "Motion," paragraph 1

46. b. Chapter 13, question 3

47. a. Chapter 12, "Background Physics and Instrumentation," end of first paragraph. Although axial resolution may be as small as 0.5 mm (1 line pair/mm), lateral resolution is 1–2 mm (3 line pairs/cm).

48. b. Chapter 12, "Problem 2"

49. c. Figure 3.15

50. c. Chapter 7, "Anode Materials," paragraph 1

INDEX

Page numbers followed by "t" denote tables; those followed by "f" denote figures.